The School-Age Child Who Stutters:
Working Effectively with Attitudes and Emotions

... A WORKBOOK

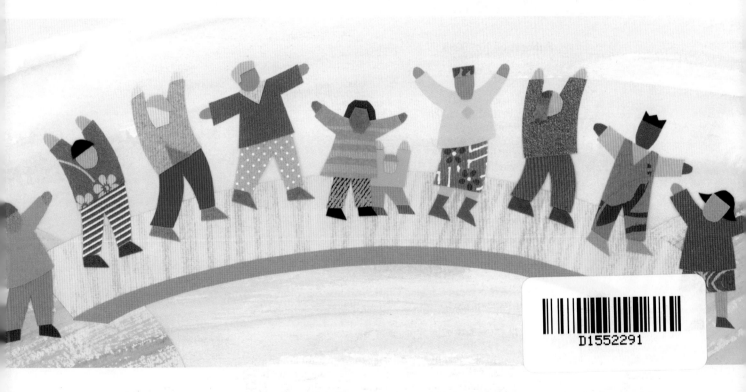

by Kristin A. Chmela, M.A., CCC-SLP
and Nina Reardon, M.S., CCC-SLP

Edited by Lisa A. Scott, Ph.D., CCC-SLP

Reproducing Pages from This Book

As described below, some of the pages in this book may be reproduced for instructional use (not for resale). To protect your book, make a photocopy of each reproducible page. Then use that copy as a master for photocopying.

the school-age child who stutters:
working effectively with attitudes and emotions

Publication No. 0005

First Edition – 2001
Second Printing – 2002
Third Printing – 2005
Fourth Printing – 2009
Fifth Printing – 2012
Sixth Printing – 2016

Published by

Stuttering Foundation of America
P.O. Box 11749
Memphis, Tennessee 38111-0749

Library of Congress Catalog Card Number: 99-71368
ISBN 0-933388-49-7

The Stuttering Foundation of America is a nonprofit charitable organization dedicated to the prevention and treatment of stuttering.

INDEX

How do attitudes and emotions fit into stuttering therapy?

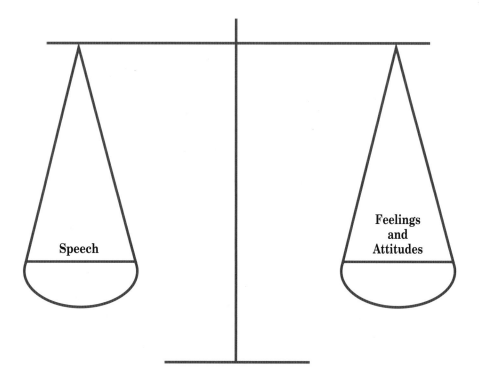

The goal of therapy is to assist children in finding the balance between...

Feeling good about talking, stuttering, and themselves

and

Being able to understand and use speech modification techniques

in order to become...

effective communicators

Chapter 1

introduction

Striking a Balance

Feelings and beliefs about stuttering, communication, and oneself are as important a part of the stuttering problem for a school-age child as the disfluency itself. We believe the goal of stuttering therapy with school-age children should be to help them become the best communicators they can be.

Teaching the child speech tools to improve fluency and change stuttering are part of improving communication skills. If he is reluctant to use those tools in front of others, still feels shame or fear when stuttering, or has difficulty solving problems like teasing, then increasing that child's fluency will not be enough. It is our job to assist the child in finding a balance between modifying speech on the one hand and developing and maintaining healthier attitudes and feelings on the other.

The Variability of Attitudes and Feelings

Because stuttering is a complex problem, the feelings and beliefs that accompany it are also complex and different for each child. Therefore, it is important to avoid making the assumption that all children who stutter will feel the same things in the same ways. There are three important points to remember when thinking about how feelings and beliefs can vary among children who stutter.

First, **the amount and type of stuttering may not be in direct relationship to the presence of negative feelings and beliefs the child is experiencing**. That is, one child may exhibit a high frequency of stuttering with many long, tense blocks, but may not feel intense negative feelings or believe he or she has poor communication skills. Another child may exhibit only mild stuttering but may feel shame and embarrassment about the problem.

For example, eight-year-old Tina demonstrated severe stuttering with many prolongations and tense blocks. However, she never avoided talking and demonstrated healthy attitudes about her speech problem and herself in general. On the other hand, Mike, aged 12, exhibited only mild stuttering but had significant negative feelings and beliefs about stuttering, communication, and himself. He told us that he was afraid and ashamed of his stuttering and avoided speech blocks by choosing not to talk at all.

Second, **children and families differ in the way they think and feel about stuttering**. Kagan (1981) suggested that some children are born with greater sensitivity to uncomfortable and unfamiliar experiences. Therefore, it's likely that children will differ in their sensitivity to listener reactions or to their own disfluencies.

If a child has greater sensitivity to listener reactions, though, he may be more likely to develop ways to hide the problem. Furthermore, he may feel fear and anxiety when using speech tools in front of others. This can be true even when use of the tools facilitates increased fluency.

For example, Drew, age 9, was skilled at using speech modification tools to improve his fluency but never used them outside the therapy room. When we explored this with him, he shared that some classmates had imitated his new speech patterns. Using tools was embarrassing to Drew because he was teased, so he chose not to use them and also to avoid talking.

Parents and teachers also have different thoughts and feelings about stuttering. The way that stuttering is perceived and talked about differs greatly from one family or classroom to another. Some families or teachers have a high degree of tolerance for stuttering and will discuss it openly with the child. Others never talk about it or have unrealistic expectations for fluency. Recognizing this variability in sensitivity can help you begin to understand how children, families, or teachers might have very different feelings and beliefs about stuttering.

Third, **children vary in their ability to understand and talk about their feelings and beliefs**. Some children may be quite open about their feelings and beliefs in the initial evaluation, while others may need support and guidance from you before they are ready, able, and willing to share their feelings and beliefs.

During one evaluation, we asked eight-year-old David if he knew why he was there. He leaned forward and said, "Would you like me to fill you in on my problem?" David went on to share that he knew he stuttered and felt that his mom was more frustrated by it than he was.

In another evaluation, we asked twelve-year-old Wesley how he felt about stuttering and he said it didn't bother him. About a month after therapy had started, we asked him to write one question he had about stuttering and bring it to the next session. Wesley wrote, "When will I quit stuttering? I hate it and want to know when I'll quit." It takes time for some children to be willing to share their attitudes and feelings.

Remembering that each child will have individual feelings, beliefs, and ability to talk about stuttering is critical to understanding the complexity of the child's problem. Perhaps even more important, though, is not making an assumption about the degree of negative feelings and beliefs based on the severity of the child's stuttering.

Examining our own role in helping the child cope with and develop more positive feelings and beliefs is another key aspect of helping children become the best communicators possible.

The Role of the Clinician

Our ability to relate effectively to each child is the foundation for helping children make changes in feelings and beliefs. Many authors have written that successful stuttering therapy depends on the quality of the clinician-client relationship (Gregory, 1991; Manning, 1996; Shapiro, 1999; Van Riper, 1958; and others).

Why is the quality of our relationship with children so important? Any person who spends time with a child will influence that child's self-image. Briggs (1975) wrote that a child's self-esteem is the most likely aspect of development that determines how the child uses his own special set of skills and abilities. Clinicians also play a critical role in "mirroring" for a child new ways in which to see himself. Children draw conclusions about themselves by comparing themselves to others and also by others' responses to them. Coopersmith (1967) found that self-esteem was best predicted by the quality of the relationship the child had with his parents rather than by wealth, education, social class, or parental occupation.

Because we spend time with children talking about experiences that are significantly related to their self-esteem, such as their willingness to talk with friends or how they respond to teasing, we have a unique opportunity to enhance their self-esteem. To make changes in stuttering, it is essential to create a relationship with a child where positive self-esteem can be developed and/or maintained.

Recognizing the variability in attitudes and feelings and the role that we have in incorporating these aspects into treatment is important to successful intervention. Although many clinicians have shared with us that they feel uncomfortable dealing with these aspects of stuttering therapy, we strongly believe that **all** clinicians can help children develop or maintain healthier attitudes and feelings about stuttering, communication, and themselves.

The Purpose of this Book

As we began our careers, we found that practical strategies for helping children who stutter change their feelings and beliefs about stuttering were almost nonexistent. As we worked with these children, we also discovered that they were not using the skills they'd learned in therapy in other environments or were experiencing significant relapses in their fluency. When we began to explore the reasons for lack of transfer or for relapse, we often traced it back to negative feelings or inaccurate beliefs the children had about stuttering and themselves as communicators.

Also, we observed that some children made marked improvement in their feelings and beliefs about stuttering. For example, they may have increased their participation in the classroom or figured out the steps to overcoming a feared speaking situation, but we struggled with methods for documenting these important treatment outcomes. As a result, we began developing tools for assessing feelings and beliefs that would help us identify any needed treatment goals.

We also needed strategies to use in treatment that would help us help children make changes. At the same time, it was important to us that the products of assessment and treatment would help document changes in feelings and beliefs as they occurred.

The purpose of this book is to provide information about assessing, documenting, and integrating attitudes and feelings as part of stuttering therapy. Although they are equally important, this book does not address specific fluency shaping and stuttering modification techniques used to help children make changes in speech behavior. A number of resources on this topic are listed in the reference section of the book.

In this first chapter, we've reviewed three things: the importance of finding a balance in treatment between working on speech and incorporating attitudes and feelings; understanding the variability of attitudes and feelings; and, our role as the clinician.

In Chapter Two, we will present strategies for improving our ability to relate to children and others. Specifically, we'll share how to validate children's feelings and respond to them using encouraging praise. We'll discuss the importance of these skills as well as why they are especially important to stuttering therapy.

In Chapter Three, we will offer you a protocol for investigating children's attitudes and feelings about themselves, communication, and stuttering. You will find pencil-paper tasks we've developed to elicit information from children, parents, and others. For each task, you will find a description, instructions for use, suggested age ranges, and available alternatives. Included in this section are examples of actual responses children have given and our perceptions of the information they have shared.

In Chapter Four, we will present nine different strategies that help children develop or maintain positive attitudes and feelings. Examples of using these strategies with children are offered. All strategies are described, including instructions for using them and sample documentation of short-term objectives. These are provided to assist you in better documenting and measuring the child's progress related to this aspect of therapy.

Finally, we will present several clinical examples in Chapter Five. In this chapter you will find case histories, assessment data, and examples of strategies used in the treatment of four children. We hope this section will help you better understand the process of assessing and integrating this aspect of stuttering into therapy.

Chapter 2

becoming better communicators

The relationship between the clinician, child, and others has been said to be the key to successful stuttering therapy (Gregory, 1991). This ability to relate depends largely upon our own communication skills. In their book, *How to Talk So Kids Will Listen and Listen So Kids Will Talk,* Faber and Mazlish (1980) discuss the process of validating children's feelings and using encouraging versus evaluative praise. Improving our ability to use these skills in stuttering therapy will most likely improve our ability to relate to the children that we work with.

Validating Children's Feelings

Children who stutter have been shown to have negative attitudes towards communication (DeNil & Brutten, 1991). When healthy expression of these attitudes is not encouraged, children may attempt to resist negative feelings as they experience them. This "resistance" may lead to physical tension (Briggs, 1975). In turn, this tension may interfere with a child's ability to successfully manage stuttering (Murphy, 1996).

When we create opportunities for children to express negative feelings and they are accepted without judgment, the negative feelings lose their destructive power (Briggs, 1975). This helps to diminish tension and may result in positive changes in how the child learns to cope with the stuttering problem. Validating feelings in this way creates a climate that encourages the child to continue to share beliefs and feelings about himself and his stuttering. Experiencing acceptance leads to a trusting clinical relationship. Subsequently, the child feels safe in attempting new behaviors and expressing himself in a more honest way.

Learning to validate a child's feelings involves a five step process.

VALIDATING FEELINGS

The child says, "I hate talking in science.
Sometimes my teacher calls on me and I don't want to answer."

Step 1: **Actively listen by acknowledging with a word.**

Clinician: **"Hmm" "Oh?" "I see."** or **"Really?"** and then wait for the child to continue talking.

Step 2: **Periodically reflect the child's message.**

Clinician: **"So what you're saying is** you hate talking in science because your teacher calls on you and you don't want to answer?"

Step 3: **Probe for more information.**

Clinician: "And you don't like talking in science **because...**" or, **"I wonder what you mean by** you don't like talking in science."

Child: "I don't like talking in science because I get into big speech blocks and the other kids laugh at me."

Step 4: **Label the feeling.**

Clinician: **"Boy, that must feel frustrating."**

(Children will quickly tell you if the feeling labeled is not correct, e.g., "No, it's not frustrating, it just makes me mad.")

Step 5: **Validate the emotion.**

Clinician: **"It's ok to feel** mad about talking in science."

Using this skill effectively often leads to a greater understanding of the child's experiences and perceptions. This leads to a clearer understanding of what they're feeling. It is important to remember that these steps don't always happen in a sequential order. That is, during a conversation you may find yourself doing a lot of reflecting and probing with the child before you get to the point where you're ready to label and validate.

Consider the following examples, first related to everyday life, then to stuttering.

VALIDATING FEELINGS
Example 1: RAUL'S STORY

Conversation A: Not Validating

Raul:	"I had the worst school day ever."
Parent:	"What happened?"
Raul:	"It's Mrs. Jones. She's too mean-she gives too much homework."
Parent:	"In middle school, you get lots of homework. That's part of growing up."

Conversation B: Validating Feelings

Raul:	"I had the worst school day ever."
Parent:	"Oh, I see. Hmm. *(active listening)* I'm wondering what the worst school day ever would be like." *(reflecting and probing)*
Raul:	"Mrs. Jones is mean. She isn't helpful at all. She throws these ridiculous assignments at us with hardly any time to do them."
Parent:	"She gave you an assignment with hardly any time to complete it? You're not finding her to be a very helpful teacher, huh?" *(reflecting and probing)*
Raul:	"That's right. She expects us to figure these problems out on our own."
Parent:	"That must feel very frustrating." *(labeling)*
Raul:	"It really is. It makes me really mad."
Parent:	"It's OK to feel mad about that." *(validating)*

In Conversation A, Raul's parent did not use communication skills that acknowledged his true concern, nor did he label and validate what Raul was feeling.

In Conversation B, the steps for validating were used and Raul's parent further understood the frustration and anxiety he was experiencing in becoming a more independent learner.

VALIDATING FEELINGS
Example 2: JONATHAN'S STORY

Conversation A: Not Validating

Clinician: "How did you like going to your previous therapy?"

Jonathan: "I sort of liked going. We played games and it was fun. But it was really pointless. She would always stop me. Even if I made the tiniest mistake. She would stop me to do it smoother and slower. I could never get anywhere!"

Clinician: "Well she was probably trying to help you. I'll bet she probably wanted you to work on your tools. Speech can be fun but it can also be work as well."

Conversation B: Validating Feelings

Clinician: "How did you like going to your previous therapy?"

Jonathan: "I sort of liked going. We played games and it was fun."

Clinician: "Oh, I see. *(active listening)* Well, speech can be fun. You sound like you really liked going." *(reflective listening)*

Jonathan: "But it was really pointless. She would always stop me."

Clinician: "You're saying it was pointless, going to speech. I'm wondering what 'pointless' means." *(reflecting and probing)*

Jonathan: "If I made the tiniest mistake, she would always stop me to do it again smoother and slower! I could never get anywhere!"

Clinician: "So she would stop you as you were talking and ask you to do it over again?" *(reflecting and probing)*

Jonathan: "Yeah that's right. I didn't want to go there anymore. I didn't like that. I wasn't allowed to make any mistakes."

Clinician: "That must have felt frustrating!" *(labeling)*

Jonathan: "No, not frustrating. It was annoying!"

Clinician: "Boy that must have been annoying! It's ok to feel annoyed by that." *(validating)*

In Conversation A, the clinician reflects her own perspective rather than probing for more information and seeking to understand Jonathan's experience.

In Conversation B, the clinician probes and Jonathan provides additional information. As they talk, he corrects her when she labels the feeling. Then, she successfully validates the child's emotion. Jonathan demonstrated an interesting perspective regarding his previous therapy. Further exploration with his previous clinician revealed her perception that Jonathan did not allow himself to make mistakes. Understanding this was an important part of determining how to approach his therapy. By using the validating process, we were able to gain additional insight into some of his attitudes and feelings.

VALIDATING FEELINGS
Example 3: GRACE'S STORY

Conversation A: Not Validating
(Child enters the room crying)

Clinician: "What's wrong?"

Grace: "It's my stuttering. It's just so hard."

Clinician: "Don't worry. It's going to get better. Look at all the progress you've made so far!"

Conversation B: Validating Feelings

Clinician: "You seem really sad today. *(observing)* Tears are OK here." *(validating)*

Grace: "It's my stuttering. It's just so hard."

Clinician: "Oh I see. *(active listening)* So it's your stuttering. It's just a tough problem to deal with, huh?" *(reflecting and probing)*

Grace: "It really is and I'm really sick of it and I wish I could wake up one day and it would be gone."

Clinician: "You must feel pretty sad." *(labeling)*

Grace: "Yeah, I do. Totally."

Clinician: "It's OK to feel sad about your stuttering." *(validating)*

In Conversation A, Grace does not feel heard. Her feelings are not labeled and accepted.

In Conversation B, the clinician creates an opportunity for Grace to express her feelings. This models for Grace the importance of communicating negative feeling and learning to accept them.

It is clear from these examples that the way in which we respond to children helps determine our ability to understand their experiences. This ultimately affects our ability to relate to the child, as well as to create and maintain a trusting relationship. It also models for the child, parents, and others better ways to listen, reflect, probe, label, and validate someone else's experience.

Using Encouraging Praise

Using encouraging praise allows us to respond to the child in ways that build positive self-esteem and create new beliefs about stuttering. Differences between praise that evaluates and praise that encourages are summarized in the chart below, Faber and Mazlish (1980).

By habit, many of us use evaluative praise. Praise of this type communicates a *value judgment* about performance. Encouraging praise, on the other hand, is simply making an *observation about behavior* and then stating how that behavior makes you feel. When you provide a label for the behavior, the child walks away with a new verbal "snapshot" of himself. Thus, our response to the child creates a window that helps the child change how he thinks about communication.

Chart 2.0: Evaluative versus Encouraging Praise	
Evaluative Praise	**Encouraging Praise**
Includes words such as great, wonderful, terrific, super	Includes description of effort or behavior
Provides judgment based on correct responses	Recognizes effort and improvement
Expresses adult's values and opinions	Can be expressed when the child isn't doing well, even if facing failure
Increases dependence on others for approval	Teaches self-motivation, belief in oneself
May create anxiety or confusion when praise does not match child's self-perceptions	Allows child to form an internal evaluation

There are three steps for providing encouraging praise to children, Faber and Mazlish (1980):

ENCOURAGING PRAISE

Step 1: **Make an observation using phrases.**
e.g., "I see that you..." "I was noticing that..." or "You were telling me that ..."
Example: "I see that you got a B+ on your math test."

Step 2: **Share how it makes you feel.**
Example: "When you get a grade you've worked hard for, I feel proud."

Step 3: **Sum it up with a word.**
Example: "You are learning how to study on your own. You are becoming independent about your school work."

Encouraging praise can also be used when things aren't going well. Watching a child struggle through math homework and saying, "Boy, math seems tough for you. You're really putting forth good effort," encourages them because you are recognizing how hard they are working even though the subject is difficult. Responding to a child who has struggled through a speech block by saying, "Boy, that was tough. Good for you for finishing," is using encouraging praise.

The following examples illustrate the use of encouraging praise in general, and then related to stuttering.

ENCOURAGING PRAISE
Example 1: JENNY

Dialogue A: Evaluative Praise

Jenny: "Here's my picture from art class, Mom."

Mom: "It's beautiful. You did a great job."

Jenny: *(Walks away thinking to herself...)* "She says that about every picture I do."

Dialogue B: Encouraging Praise

Jenny: "Here's my picture from art class, Mom."

Mom: "Wow! I see you used the colors green, yellow, and blue and that you blended them with a special sponge. *(describing what she sees with detail)* The design in this picture makes me feel happy when I look at it. *(stating how it makes her feel)* Jenny, you are really artistic!" *(summing it up with a word)*

Jenny: *(Walks away thinking to herself...)* "Boy, I am really artistic!"

ENCOURAGING PRAISE
Example 2: SUSIE

At the beginning of a therapy session, thirteen-year-old Susie tells her clinician a story and exhibits some tense speech blocks. This type of stuttering had not been previously observed by the clinician. Susie had shared that she felt her stuttering was "bad" and that she hides it most of the time.

Evaluative Praise

Following the tense speech block, the clinician might say nothing or say: "Let's try that one again only a little smoother."

Encouraging Praise

Following the tense speech block, the clinician says: "Susie I was noticing that you've been getting pretty tense on some of your words. *(describing the behavior)*
Actually, that was great stuttering. I am honored you would share it with me and let me see what it looks like. *(stating how it makes the clinician feel)* Stuttering is OK. You decided not to hide it. You are really courageous." *(summing it up with a word)*

ENCOURAGING PRAISE
Example 3: NICK

Nick, a fifth grader, comes to the therapy room in middle school and announces that he stood up in front of the class and gave a short speech.

Dialogue A: Evaluative Praise

Nick: "I got up in front of the class today and talked and I didn't even stutter."

Clinician: "Great job, Nick. That was just great. I knew you could do it."

Dialogue B: Encouraging Praise

Nick: "I got up in front of the class today and talked and I didn't even stutter."

Clinician: "Nick, you say you got up in front of the class and gave a talk just like the rest of the kids? *(describing the behavior)* I feel proud that you felt comfortable enough to do that. *(stating how it makes her feel).* Your contribution to the class is very important. You are really brave!" *(summing it up with a word)*

ENCOURAGING PRAISE
Example 4: JOEY

The clinician observes Joey using easy speech on his own as he enters the therapy room.

Evaluative Praise

Clinician: "That was great smooth speech, Joey!"

Encouraging Praise

Clinician: "Joey, I just heard you use your easy speech when you came in the room. *(describing the behavior)* I feel excited that you're changing your speech on your own *(stating how it makes her feel)* You are really a smart thinker about speech tools!" *(summing it up with a word)*

Often, the language we use when we encourage children directly reflects the goals we want children to achieve in therapy. If we want children to become open, responsible, and capable of managing their stuttering, then the language we use to encourage them reflects those goals. If we want children to stop avoiding stuttering, we can encourage them for being courageous and letting the stuttering happen. Opportunities for offering encouraging praise often occur after validating the child's feelings, as in the next example.

VALIDATING AND ENCOURAGING COMBINED: JOSH'S STORY

Josh: "I made a phone call today and I couldn't say my name. The mother hung up on me."

Clinician: "Oh....... Really........ *(actively listening)* You say you made a phone call and couldn't get the word out. *(reflecting and probing)* That must have been frustrating." *(labeling the feeling)*

Josh: "Yeah. It was. But I just picked up the phone and tried to call again."

Clinician: "Oh...... *(actively listening)* You called back?" *(reflecting and probing)*

Josh: "Yeah I did and when his mom answered I finally got out who I was. Then I told her that I stuttered a lot on the phone and that it was me that had called before."

Clinician: "So you told her what happened when you called the first time?" *(reflecting)*

Josh: "I did, and she told me she was sorry that she hung up. I told her it was OK and that sometimes people do that because they don't know the person that is calling is in a block."

Clinician: "You were able to explain to her what had happened, then. *(reflecting)* Wow. You know, when you do something like that I feel proud of you! (*sharing how it makes her feel)* First, you came in today and shared this experience with me. Second, you had the courage to make the phone call and then when it was tough, you picked up the phone and called again! And, you shared with the mom what had happened! *(describing the behaviors with detail)* You are taking responsibility for your speech problem!" *(summing it up with a word)*

Teaching these communication skills to parents and teachers will increase their understanding of the child's experiences. When a child who stutters is surrounded by adults who validate and offer encouraging praise, the child's expression of feelings is supported; and we can make greater progress in therapy.

Chapter 3

assessment

A comprehensive assessment of a child's stuttering includes obtaining a thorough case history, documenting frequency and severity of the stuttering behavior, and examining other communication skills such as language and phonology. It also includes discovering others' perceptions of the communication problem (i.e., parents and teachers), as well as assessing the child's attitudes and feelings about stuttering. Given the purpose of this book, strategies useful in assessing attitudes and feelings will be presented. If you need more information regarding comprehensive evaluation of stuttering, the reference list at the end of this book contains a number of helpful resources.

Assessing attitudes and feelings in regards to stuttering is an essential part of the screening process and evaluation. The information we get from children about their perceptions and knowledge of the problem is critical for treatment planning. This is especially true when the child does not stutter openly in your therapy room. In our experience, children who attempt to hide or cover up their stuttering are often the ones who have negative attitudes and feelings related to the problem.

Therefore, we want to explore the following:

1. How does the child see the problem?
    a. Is he aware of the problem?
    b. How does he describe the speech difficulty?
    c. What does he call the problem ("stuttering," "bumpy speech," "hard talking")?

2. What is the child's level of concern?
    a. How worried does he appear to be about the stuttering?
    b. Does he express concern to others?

3. Is the child working to hide the stuttering?
   a. Does he use word substitutions?
   b. Does he avoid certain situations or words?
   c. Does he describe fears related to talking?

4. How do others (e.g., parents and teachers) see the problem?
   a. Do others think the child is concerned about the problem?
   b. Why do they think the child is concerned?
   c. What are their concerns?

We have formed perceptions about this information by using the following protocol: general questions, specific questions, and paper-pencil tasks. Standardized scales, such as the **Children's Attitudes About Talking-Revised** (DeNil & Brutten, 1991) or the **A-19 Scale** (Andre & Guitar, 1991) can also be used.

How to Talk With Children About Talking

Forming a positive clinician-child relationship begins at the screening and evaluation stages. At the initiation of either process, it is critical for clinicians to show an interest in what the *child* is interested in and to structure an initial activity that is enjoyable to him. This allows the clinician to relate positively to the child and creates an opportunity to begin talking about talking. We often play a game or complete an art project at the start of our interactions.

Earlier in our careers, we used to ask children the direct question "How do you feel about your speech?" One of three answers were usually given: (1)"Fine," (2) "I don't know," or (3) they said nothing. As a result, we developed the following protocol to elicit this information from children.

During an enjoyable activity, we begin talking with the child about their special interests, such as pets, sports, or hobbies. As the child becomes comfortable, we start exploring their attitudes and feelings about their talking with *general* questions. For example:

➤ "Do you like talking?"

➤ "Who do you like to talk to the best?"

- ➤ "What do you like to talk about the most?"

- ➤ "Is talking usually easy for you?"

- ➤ "If you could change something about your talking, what would it be?"

- ➤ "Do you know why you're here today?"

We listen carefully to how the child describes the problem. Some children may discuss communication difficulties in general terms, such as "I talk too fast," while others may use more descriptive terms. Some children may say, "Talking is hard," "I don't like talking," "I'm here because I stutter," or "I want to change how my speech comes out." Others may indicate no awareness at all. The language **the child uses** to answer our questions becomes **the language we use** to talk about the problem (Williams, 1985).

The child's responses to these general questions help us determine what to ask next. If, at this point, the child demonstrates no awareness of the problem, we don't question further. However, if something the child says suggests they are aware, we continue with further probing.

Questions that probe further into more specific attitudes and feelings about stuttering may include:

- ➤ "What does that mean?" e.g., "What does that mean, stuttering?" or "What is that, bumpy speech?"

- ➤ "What about your speech do you want to change?"

- ➤ "What does it look like/sound like?"

- ➤ "When does it happen?"

- ➤ "Who does it happen with?"

- ➤ "What do you do when it happens?"

- ➤ "Do you know why it happens?"

- ➤ "Has anyone ever said anything to you about your speech?"

➤ "Is there anything you do to make it better/easier?"

➤ "Does it ever make you feel ... happy, sad, mad, frustrated?"

➤ "How did you get so smart about this?"

Notice the different responses children might have to these questions as illustrated in Chart 3.0. These are actual questions and responses taken directly from evaluation transcripts.

Chart 3.0: Examples of Further Probing	
Clinician's Question	**Child's Response**
"Is there anything about your talking you'd like to change?" "What do you mean, the way you stutter?" "What do you do when it happens?"	*B., age 10:* "I'd like to change the way I stutter." *B.:* "It's when I get really excited about an idea and the words don't come out." *B.:* "I try not to stutter by slowing down but the kids at school tell me I'm weird when I do that."
"Hi Mike, it's nice to meet you," as he entered the room.	*M., age 13:* "I'm a stutterer. There are days I just can't talk." (He got right to the point!)
"Do you like to talk?" "What does that mean, 'bumpy'?" "Does it ever make you feel mad or frustrated?" "Is there anything you do that makes your speech 'not bumpy'?"	*L., age 8:* "Yes, I do. But sometimes when I talk, my voice gets bumpy." *L.:* "Like when I say oooo ppenn" *L.:* "I get mad when it happens because nobody else's voice is like mine." *L.:* "I don't talk."

These dialogues are documented as part of the evaluation data. They are shared with parents and teachers and help illustrate the impact attitudes and feelings can have on a stuttering problem.

The Use of Paper-Pencil Tasks

In our experience, children often give us information through writing that they may not share in conversation. Therefore, when appropriate, we follow up these discussions by administering selected paper-pencil tasks. Choosing two, three, or more appropriate tasks can provide important additional information. The tasks are chosen based on (a) the child's age, (b) cognitive ability, and (c) awareness of the problem. These paper-pencil tasks are not only useful at the evaluation but also during the therapy process to document changes in attitudes and feelings over time.

Children's responses give us insight into how they feel about themselves, communication, and stuttering. Although highly subjective, we believe these tasks provide critical information in helping us, the child's parents, and teachers understand the child's perception of the problem. In general, we look for information about the following:

> ➤ How do they feel about themselves in general?

> ➤ Do they include stuttering in any of their responses?

> ➤ How does stuttering compare to other things the child includes in their responses?

> ➤ What aspects about communication are mentioned in relation to the family, peers, and others?

Chart 3.1 provides a summary of the paper-pencil tasks we have developed. It includes suggested age ranges and brief descriptions for each. Following this chart, each paper-pencil task is provided. We have included actual examples of each task from children with our comments on their responses. Many paper-pencil tasks are similar in nature. Therefore, use your knowledge of the child to determine which tasks are most appropriate.

Chart 3.1: Summary of Paper-Pencil Tasks

Task	Suggested Age Ranges	Description
What's True for You?	8 and older	Classifying statements about stuttering on a 7-point rating scale
Here's What I Think	9 and older	Open-ended questions regarding previous stuttering therapy
My Views on School	8 and older	Open-ended questions regarding talking at school
Hands Down	8 and older	Listing of positive/negative attributes
Write a Word Picture	8 and older	Listing of positive/negative attributes
Important Stuff	10 years and older	List of important information child wants to share about self
What Pops?	9 and older	Sentence completion task
Count Me Out	12 and older	Scaling avoidance of certain speaking situations
Worry Ladder	9 and older	Listing "worries" in rank order
Framing My Speech	10 and older	Selecting words that describe feelings regarding stuttering
Draw Me A Picture	5 and older	Self-portraits on "easy" and "hard" speech days
My Family and I	6 and older	A drawing of the child with his/her family
How I See My Stuttering	9 and older	Drawing a picture representing feelings regarding stuttering
Parent Questionnaire	Parents	Open-ended statements regarding parents' perceptions of the probem
Teacher Questionnaire	Teachers	Open-ended statements regarding teacher's perceptions of the probem

The attitudes and feelings a child "brings" to our table about stuttering are directly related to the goals we develop. While some children need to develop healthier attitudes and feelings about stuttering and self, our goal for other children may be to assist them in maintaining their positive attitudes and feelings.

Furthermore, remember that attitudes and feelings are constantly changing over time. Our clinical experience has shown that as children learn to change speech behaviors, they begin to feel better about talking. Likewise, as children learn more about the problem (i.e., change attitudes), they are better able to make changes in how they are talking.

For some children, as their own awareness as well as peer awareness increases, they may become more sensitive about how they speak. Also, during periods of relapse, we may notice attitudes and feelings that become more negative. Therefore, continuing to explore and document the child's attitudes and feelings *throughout* therapy is important. In addition, treatment should include goals that address changes as they are noted.

Paper-Pencil Task #1:
What's True For You?

DESCRIPTION/PURPOSE:

This paper-pencil task uses a 7-point rating scale to gain information about the child's perception of talking.

WHEN & HOW TO USE:

We use this with most children, especially those who have verbalized an awareness of their stuttering problem.

SPECIAL INSTRUCTIONS/NOTES:

We recommend that this task be administered orally as an interview guide. If the child provides information that is unclear or that suggests the need for further probing, you can continue to explore the topic throughout the interview.

AN ALTERNATIVE PAPER-PENCIL TASK:

None.

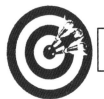

WHAT'S TRUE FOR YOU?

Name:_____

Date:_____

Age:_____

Read each statement. Circle the number that best describes what's true for you.

1. I wish I could talk like other kids.

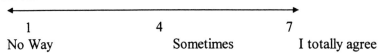

1	4	7
No Way	Sometimes	I totally agree

2. Some people are hard to talk to.

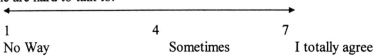

1	4	7
No Way	Sometimes	I totally agree

3. I talk openly about my speech with my parents.

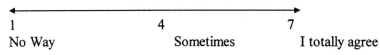

1	4	7
No Way	Sometimes	I totally agree

4. I am a good talker.

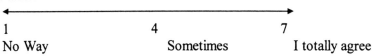

1	4	7
No Way	Sometimes	I totally agree

5. I like to talk.

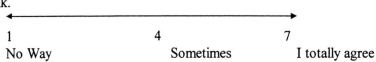

1	4	7
No Way	Sometimes	I totally agree

6. Sometimes I do things so I won't have trouble talking (like not talking or changing words or thoughts).

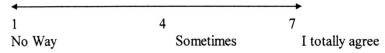

1	4	7
No Way	Sometimes	I totally agree

7. I have sounds that are hard for me to say.

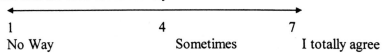

1   4   7
No Way   Sometimes   I totally agree

8. It's O.K. to have trouble talking sometimes.

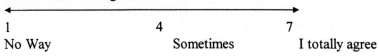

1   4   7
No Way   Sometimes   I totally agree

9. I have gotten teased about my speech.

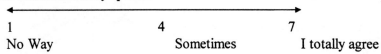

1   4   7
No Way   Sometimes   I totally agree

10. I don't like having trouble talking.

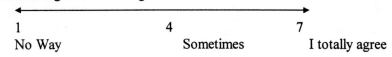

1   4   7
No Way   Sometimes   I totally agree

11. I want to improve the way I talk.

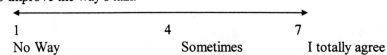

1   4   7
No Way   Sometimes   I totally agree

Appropriate for ages 8 years and older

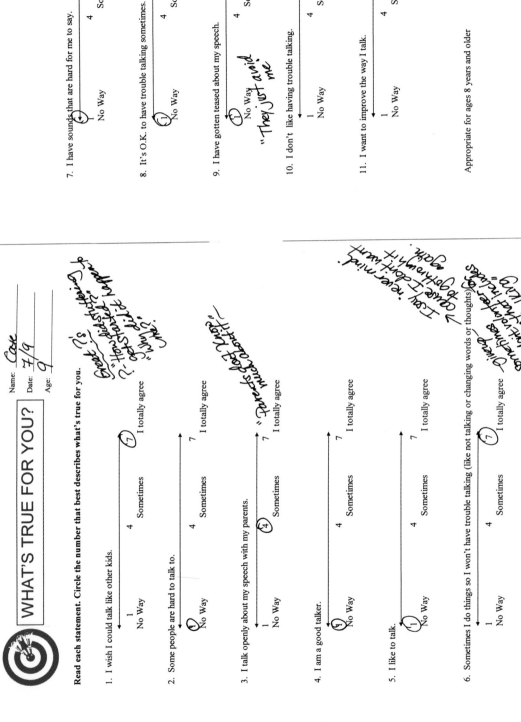

WHAT'S TRUE FOR YOU?

Name: Cate
Date: 7/9
Age: 9

Read each statement. Circle the number that best describes what's true for you.

1. I wish I could talk like other kids.

   1 No Way — 4 Sometimes — ⑦ I totally agree

   Great justification "How hard is it?" "Why?"

2. Some people are hard to talk to.

   1 No Way — 4 Sometimes — 7 I totally agree

3. I talk openly about my speech with my parents.

   1 No Way — ④ Sometimes — 7 I totally agree

   "Parents don't know"

4. I am a good talker.

   ① No Way — 4 Sometimes — 7 I totally agree

5. I like to talk.

   ① No Way — 4 Sometimes — 7 I totally agree

6. Sometimes I do things so I won't have trouble talking (like not talking or changing words or thoughts)

   1 No Way — 4 Sometimes — ⑦ I totally agree

7. I have sounds that are hard for me to say.

   ① No Way — 4 Sometimes — 7 I totally agree

8. It's O.K. to have trouble talking sometimes.

   ① No Way — 4 Sometimes — 7 I totally agree

9. I have gotten teased about my speech.

   ① No Way — 4 Sometimes — 7 I totally agree

   "They just avoid me"

10. I don't like having trouble talking.

    1 No Way — 4 Sometimes — ⑦ I totally agree

11. I want to improve the way I talk.

    1 No Way — 4 Sometimes — ⑦ I totally agree

    "Very much."

Appropriate for ages 8 years and older

CLINICIAN'S COMMENTS

Cate's example illustrates how children often make further comments based on the statements provided. She was open in her frustration with her stuttering as evidenced by the comments she made regarding avoidance. Her responses also indicated that parents and peers lacked information about stuttering. This information was important for treatment planning.

⊚ WHAT'S TRUE FOR YOU?

Name: _Justin_
Date: _1/15_
Age: _12_

Read each statement. Circle the number that best describes what's true for you.

1. I wish I could talk like other kids.

1
No Way — 4 Sometimes — ⑦ I totally agree

2. Some people are hard to talk to.

1
No Way — 4 Sometimes — ⑦ I totally agree

— Parents
— friends in the lunchroom

3. I talk openly about my speech with my parents.

① No Way — 4 Sometimes — 7 I totally agree

— we've never really talked about it

4. I am a good talker.

1
No Way — 4 Sometimes — ✗ 7 I totally agree

— pretty much

5. I like to talk.

1
No Way — 4 Sometimes — 7 I totally agree

6. Sometimes I do things so I won't have trouble talking (like not talking or changing words or thoughts).

1
No Way — 4 Sometimes — ✗ 7 I totally agree

certain words... the person... I'm going to talk to... all around

7. I have sounds that are hard for me to say.

1
No Way — ④ ✗ 4 Sometimes — 7 I totally agree

see it

8. It's O.K. to have trouble talking sometimes.

1
No Way — 4 Sometimes — ✗ ⑦ I totally agree

I guess

9. I have gotten teased about my speech.

① No Way — 4 Sometimes — 7 I totally agree

really never

10. I don't like having trouble talking.

1
No Way — 4 Sometimes — ⑦ I totally agree

11. I want to improve the way I talk.

1
No Way — 4 Sometimes — ⑦ I totally agree

yes

Appropriate for ages 8 years and older

CLINICIAN'S COMMENTS

This example is from an older child. **Justin's** responses were specific and showed he was analytical about his speech. He had excellent awareness of what was difficult for him, and suggested his parents needed to be educated about stuttering. It was also encouraging for us to note that Justin still liked talking and had positive feelings about himself.

29

Paper-Pencil Task #2:
Here's What I Think

DESCRIPTION/PURPOSE:

These open-ended questions about previous therapy yield more specific information than the child might offer when simply asked, "What did you do in speech before?" or "Did you like going to speech?" Children who report negative feelings about previous therapy indicate the need for us to be creative in how we approach therapy now.

WHEN & HOW TO USE:

Use whenever the child has previously received therapy for stuttering.

SPECIAL INSTRUCTIONS/NOTES:

We feel this instrument is best used orally in an interview with the child, although it can be completed individually by the child.

AN ALTERNATIVE PAPER-PENCIL TASK:

None.

Name:_____

Date:_____

Age:_____

Here's What I Think

1. I am here because_____

2. In previous therapy I learned _____

3. Some things I liked about my previous speech therapy were_____

_____

4. Some things I did not like about my previous speech therapy were_____

_____

5. My parents were involved in my previous therapy.   (circle one)

    Yes   No   If yes, How?_____

_____

6. I want to come to speech now   (circle one)   yes   no

    Why?_____

_____

7. A question I have about stuttering is _____

_____

8. I feel comfortable/uncomfortable (circle one) talking to my parents about my speech because

_____

Appropriate for ages 9 years and older

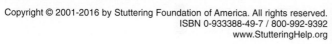

Name: Caroline
Date: 9/98
Age: 9

Here's What I Think

1. I am here because _My Mom signed me up_

2. In previous therapy I learned _sliding the words together._

3. Some things I liked about my previous speech therapy were _O_
   _____

4. Some things I did not like about my previous speech therapy were _we did_
   nothing

5. My parents were involved in my previous therapy.   (circle one)
   (Yes)   No   If yes, How? _in Kindergarten,_
   sometimes, but after that - not much.

6. I want to come to speech now   (circle one)   (yes)   no
   Why? _because I think I have a better chance of improving_
   _____

7. A question I have about stuttering is _How do I deal with stutring?_
   _____

8. I feel comfortable/(uncomfortable) (circle one) talking to my parents about my speech because
   I don't like to talk about it.

Appropriate for ages 9 years and older

CLINICIAN'S COMMENTS

Caroline reported negative feelings about past therapy but seemed to be optimistic about her current enrollment. The need for open, comfortable communication with her parents about stuttering was evident.

Here's What I Think

1. I am here because **I am a person who stutters**

2. In previous therapy I learned **how to ~~control~~ try to control my stuttering**

3. Some things I liked about my previous speech therapy were **it was fun in lower grades**

4. Some things I did not like about my previous speech therapy were **In Jr. High I was pulled out of class unexpeotidly + was asked same ?'s over and over.**

5. My parents were involved in my previous therapy.   (circle one)
   (Yes)   No   If yes, How? **They tried to talk to me about stuttering / they gave me a sign to tell me I was stuttering**

6. I want to come to speech now   (circle one)   (yes)   no
   Why? **I want to stop stuttering**

7. A question I have about stuttering is **Why me? Why do I have to go through this?**

8. I feel (comfortable) uncomfortable (circle one) talking to my parents about my speech because **I know they will be there for me no matter how bad I stutter.**

Appropriate for ages 9 years and older

CLINICIAN'S COMMENTS

Mike revealed positive aspects of previous therapy. His responses suggested further education about stuttering was needed. Finally, Mike communicated that his family was supportive and accepting of his stuttering.

Paper-Pencil Task #3:
My Views On School

DESCRIPTION/PURPOSE:

To gain information regarding how the child feels about communicating at school.

WHEN & HOW TO USE:

We typically give this instrument during an oral interview with the child, but it can be done independently.

SPECIAL INSTRUCTIONS/NOTES:

The child's responses may prompt you to explore whether the teacher's perceptions match the child's, and whether your direct observations of the child in the classroom matches the child's perceptions. Teachers have shown an interest in seeing these comments.

AN ALTERNATIVE PAPER-PENCIL TASK:

None.

Name:_____

Date:_____

Age:_____

My Views on School...

Fill in each blank with whatever comes to your mind.

1. Something I like about school is...

2. Something I don't like about school is...

3. My favorite subject in school is...

4. Places that are easy to talk in school include...

5. Places that are hard to talk in school include...

6. When I have to talk in front of the class, I feel...

7. When I'm called on to read, I feel...

8. When my teacher asks a question in class, I usually...

9. When I have trouble talking, the other kids usually...

10. My talking in the lunchroom is...

11. My talking on the playground is...

12. When I talk to adults at school, I feel...

Appropriate for ages eight and older

Name: Jill

Date: 9/19

Age: 13

My Views on School...

Fill in each blank with whatever comes to your mind.

1. Something I like about school is...
   seeing my friends

2. Something I don't like about school is...
   presentations, reading out loud in class

3. My favorite subject in school is...
   math

4. Places that are easy to talk in school include...
   on the playground/outside with my friends.

5. Places that are hard to talk in school include...
   in the classroom

6. When I have to talk in front of the class, I feel...
   very nervous

7. When I'm called on to read, I feel...
   nervous and scared that I won't be able to do a good job.

8. When my teacher asks a question in class, I usually...
   look down at my book.

9. When I have trouble talking, the other kids usually...
   Some kids will make fun of the way I talk, and others will just wait until I finish talking (my friends), some kids stare.

10. My talking in the lunchroom is...
    pretty easy - if I am not in a very big group

11. My talking on the playground is...
    pretty good

12. When I talk to adults at school, I feel...
    nervous & I worry that they won't understand what I am trying to say

Appropriate for ages eight and older

CLINICIAN'S COMMENTS

Jill's responses suggest she feels pressure to talk in the classroom and is concerned about peer responses to her stuttering. Jill's teacher confirmed that she was avoiding speaking in the classroom.

Paper-Pencil Task #4:
Hands Down

DESCRIPTION/PURPOSE:

This task elicits the child's perceptions of his positive and negative attributes.

WHEN & HOW TO USE:

This task is usually completed with younger school-age children. The child traces her own hands on a piece of paper. She lists things she likes about herself on the left hand, and things she doesn't like or wishes she could change on the right hand.

SPECIAL INSTRUCTIONS/NOTES:

This task works best at times when the child is allowed to complete it independently. Observe the child and note how long it takes her to complete the task. Is there a difference in the amount of time it takes to identify positive versus negative aspects? How many positive aspects does she list? How many negative? Does stuttering show up on either the positive or negative side? It may also be completed with the child.

AN ALTERNATIVE PAPER-PENCIL TASK:

For older children, **Write a Word Picture** or **Important Stuff** can be used.

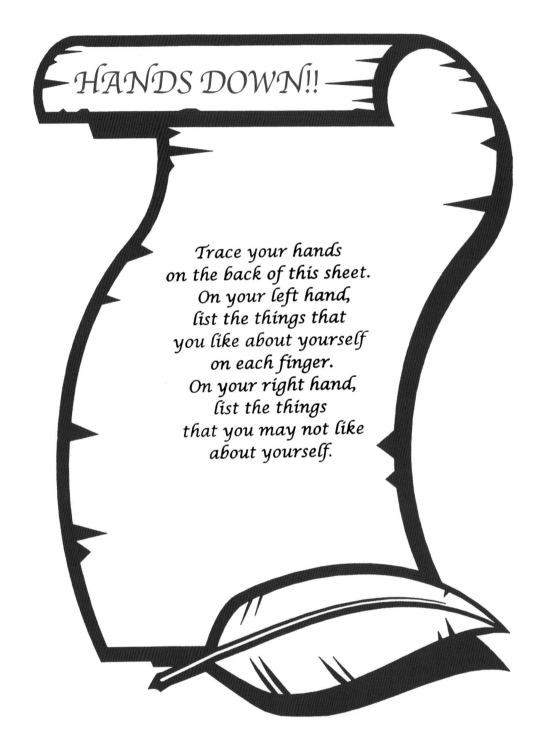

HANDS DOWN!!

Trace your hands
on the back of this sheet.
On your left hand,
list the things that
you like about yourself
on each finger.
On your right hand,
list the things
that you may not like
about yourself.

Appropriate for ages 8 years and older

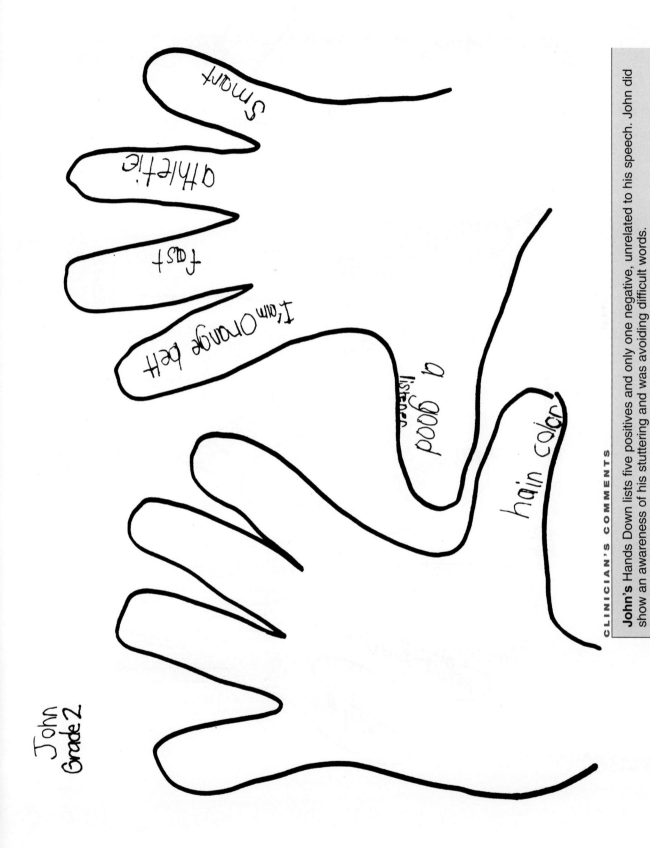

John
Grade 2

smart
athletic
fast
I am Orange belt
a good listener
hair color

CLINICIAN'S COMMENTS

John's Hands Down lists five positives and only one negative, unrelated to his speech. John did show an awareness of his stuttering and was avoiding difficult words.

Susan age 4

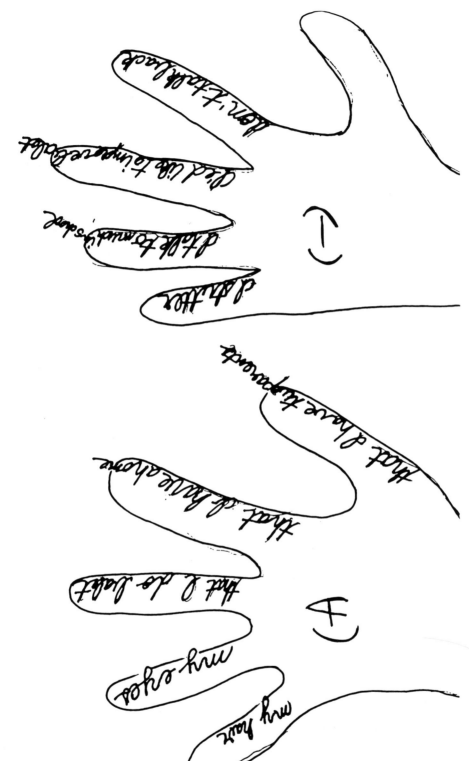

don't think back

don't like to impress people

think I'm not so smart

did her

what I have that's important

think I have a little above

that I do hair

my eyes

my hair

Susan aged 4

CLINICIAN'S COMMENTS

Susan, who overtly exhibited mild stuttering, included it on her negative hand. We had never seen her stutter in therapy, yet she rated it as one of her primary negative attributes. This suggested she had great sensitivity about her stuttering.

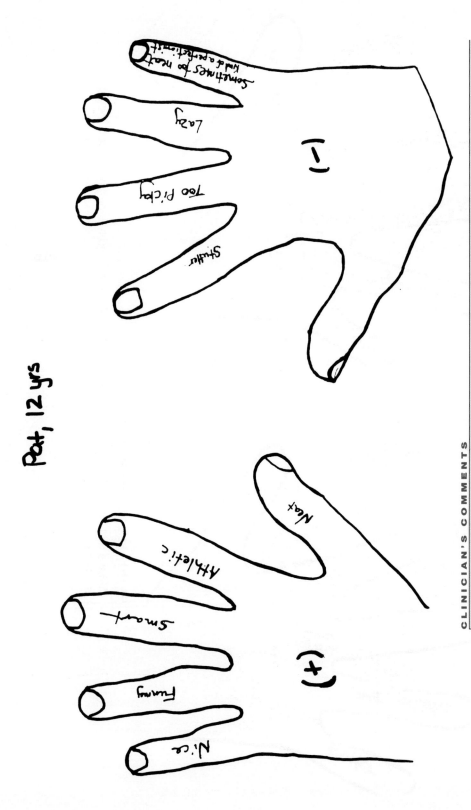

Pat, 12 yrs

(Hand tracing with labels:)
- Lazy
- Too Picky
- Sometimes too neat, kind of a perfectionist
- Shy/a
- (−)
- Neat
- Athletic
- Smart
- Funny
- Nice
- (+)

CLINICIAN'S COMMENTS

Pat's list of positive traits suggested a high self-esteem. The negatives he included suggest that he might find stuttering hard to deal with, as he is "picky" and "kind of a perfectionist." This activity increased our awareness of how he viewed his personality in addition to how he felt about his stuttering.

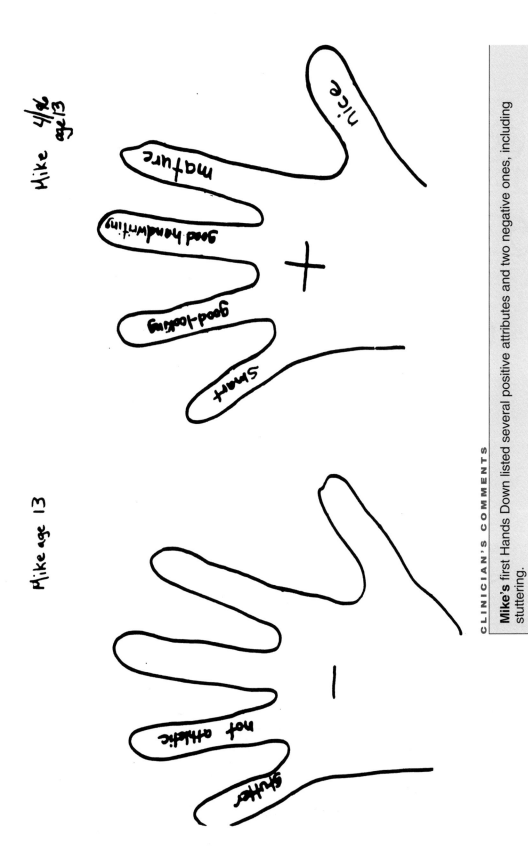

Mike 4/96
age 13

Mike age 13

nice

mature

good handwriting

good-looking

Smart

+

−

not athletic

stutter

42

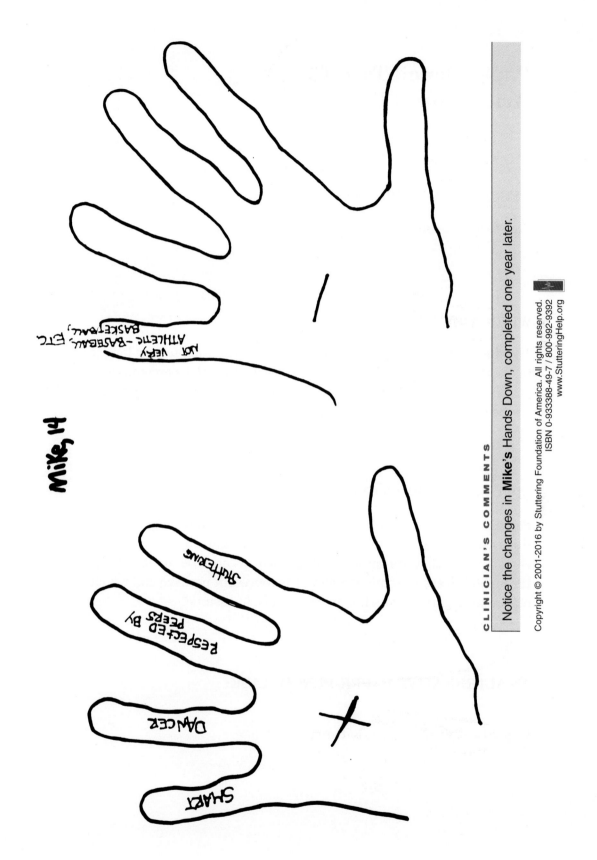

Mike, 14

NOT VERY ATHLETIC - BASEBALL, BASKETBALL, ETC.

STUTTERING

RESPECTED BY PEERS

DANCER

SMART

CLINICIAN'S COMMENTS

Notice the changes in **Mike's** Hands Down, completed one year later.

Paper-Pencil Task #5:
Write a Word Picture

DESCRIPTION/PURPOSE:

This task determines how the child describes himself.

WHEN & HOW TO USE:

This task is best completed individually. Pay attention to how long it takes the child to complete the task as well as the percentage of positive versus negative words he includes. Does stuttering show up on the list? In what order do the positive and negative words appear?

SPECIAL INSTRUCTIONS/NOTES:

Some children may need you to define "positive" and "negative." In this case, it's best if you give them examples that apply to you, the clinician, and that are rather neutral such as "athletic" or "hurried." It's helpful to ask the child which words represent positive and which represent negative traits-it's important not to assume!

AN ALTERNATIVE PAPER-PENCIL TASK:

Important Stuff or **Hands Down**

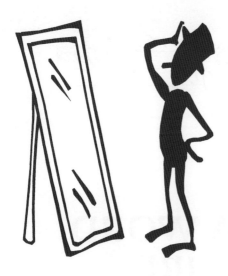

WRITE A WORD PICTURE

List on this page a series of ten words (positive or negative) that describe you.

Appropriate for ages 8 years and older

Name: Anna
Date: 8/19
Age: 9½

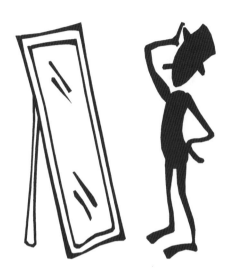

WRITE A WORD PICTURE

List on this page a series of ten words (positive or negative) that describe you.

nice, charming, humorous, young artist,
Shy around kids, some-times chatter box,
Lisa Frank Fan, stutters, 9½, 6 people in family
(Includes me) likes books.

Appropriate for ages 8 years and older

CLINICIAN'S COMMENTS

Anna included stuttering in her list, though she felt it was a positive trait. She does include more positives than negatives.

Name: Sean
Date: 10/19
Age: 11

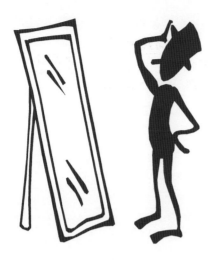

WRITE A WORD PICTURE

List on this page a series of ten words (positive or negative) that describe you.

Cool
positive
funny
Sensitive
likable
active
athletic
Popular
friendly
tricky

Appropriate for ages 8 years and older

CLINICIAN'S COMMENTS

Sean's confidence and high self-esteem are evident in this word picture.

Paper-Pencil Task #6:
Important Stuff

DESCRIPTION/PURPOSE:

Similar to **Write a Word Picture,** this task determines how the child describes himself.

WHEN & HOW TO USE:

This task is best completed individually. Pay attention to how long it takes the child to complete the task, the percentage and order of positive versus negative words they include, and whether stuttering appears.

SPECIAL INSTRUCTIONS/NOTES:

None.

AN ALTERNATIVE PAPER-PENCIL TASK:

Write a Word Picture or **Hands Down**

Name: _____

Date: _____

IMPORTANT STUFF...

...ABOUT ME!!

List things about yourself that are positive, negative, and interesting.

Positive Stuff ☺	Negative Stuff	Interesting Stuff

Appropriate for ages 10 years and older

Name: Nathan
Date: 10-11
Age: 10

IMPORTANT STUFF...
...ABOUT ME!!

List things about yourself that are positive, negative, and interesting.

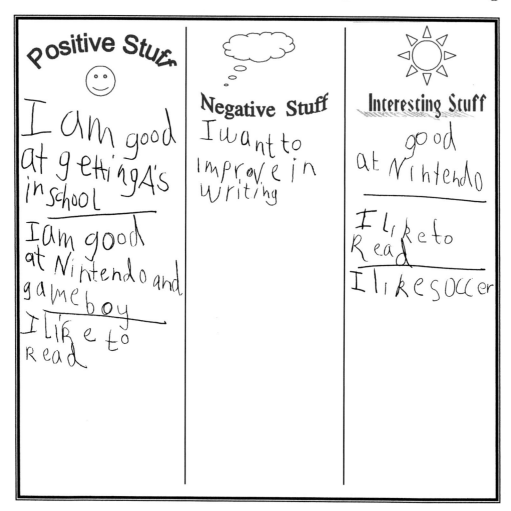

Positive Stuff 😊

I am good at getting A's in school

I am good at Nintendo and gameboy

I like to read

Negative Stuff

I want to improve in writing

Interesting Stuff

good at Nintendo

I like to Read

I like soccer

Appropriate for ages 10 years and older

CLINICIAN'S COMMENTS

Nathan quickly wrote 3 positive and 3 interesting aspects about himself. He responded to "negative stuff" last.

Name: Angela

Date: _____

IMPORTANT STUFF...
...ABOUT ME!!

List things about yourself that are positive, negative, and interesting.

Positive Stuff

I get good grades

I love to swim

I have lots of friends

I am athletic

Negative Stuff

I get headaches often

I stutter

Interesting Stuff

I collect all different kinds of music

My favorite food is deep fried oreos

Appropriate for ages 10 years and older

CLINICIAN'S COMMENTS

Angela has more positive and interesting points than negatives. She does view stuttering as a negative aspect of herself.

Paper-Pencil Task #7:
What Pops?

DESCRIPTION/PURPOSE:

This sentence completion task elicits spontaneous responses to open-ended questions.

WHEN & HOW TO USE:

This is best completed independently. Notice responses that relate to stuttering or to communication patterns within the family.

SPECIAL INSTRUCTIONS/NOTES:

None.

AN ALTERNATIVE PAPER-PENCIL TASK:

None.

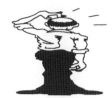

WHAT "POPS?"

...into your mind?

Name:_____

Date:_____

Age:_____

Complete the sentences below with the first thing that "pops" into your mind.
There are no right or wrong answers.

1. Most of all I want_____

2. I'm afraid_____

3. I know I can_____

4. I hate_____

5. I worry about_____

6. My family_____

7. There is nothing_____

8. I wish_____

9. Mother and I_____

10. When I get mad_____

11. At school_____

12. I want to know_____

13. I will never_____

14. My friends think I_____

15. I get mad when_____

16. My mother never_____

17. I wish my father_____

18. I just can't_____

19. I'm different because_____

20. My best friend_____

Appropriate for ages 9 years and older

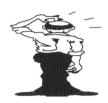

WHAT "POPS?"

...into your mind?

Name: Jamal
Date: 9/18
Age: 11

Complete the sentences below with the first thing that "pops" into your mind.
There are no right or wrong answers.

1. Most of all I want _N64_
2. I'm afraid _of killer movies_
3. I know I can _help my speech_
4. I hate _when my sisters annoy me._
5. I worry about _my grades_
6. My family _is big_
7. There is nothing _else I like but playing the snow_
8. I wish _N64 or Playstation_
9. Mother and I _play a nintendo together_
10. When I get mad _I start screaming_
11. At school _I play with friends_
12. I want to know _my grades_
13. I will never _win $_
14. My friends think I _am cool_
15. I get mad ~~when~~ _at ~~stop~~ my speech problem_
16. My mother never _stand my sisters_
17. I wish my father _and mom stop worrying ~ my speech_
18. I just can't _stand my sisters_
19. I'm different because _I have different qualities_
20. My best friend _is cool_

Appropriate for ages 9 years and older

CLINICIAN'S COMMENTS

Jamal's response on number three, "I know I can help my speech," signals a positive belief about changing stuttering. His mention of his parents' worrying about his speech (number 17) signaled a communication dynamic that warranted further exploration.

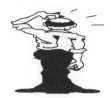

WHAT "POPS?"

...into your mind?

Name: _Caryn_
Date _5/1996_
Age: _18_

Complete the sentences below with the first thing that "pops" into your mind.
There are no right or wrong answers.

1. Most of all I want _to solve my stuttering._

2. I'm afraid _when I talk to my teachers._

3. I know I can _stopped stuttering if I try._

4. I hate _when I fight with my brother._

5. I worry about _test and school and stuttering in school. My friends get good grades and they don't stutter._

6. My family _asks me questions alot._

7. There is nothing _wrong with people who stutter._

8. I wish _I could stop stuttering._

9. Mother and I _talk alot and sometimes fight about stupid things._

10. When I get mad _I scream and yell. I never stutter when I'm mad._

11. At school _I talk alot._

12. I want to know _what made me stutter and why I do._

13. I will never _talk back to a teacher._

14. My friends think I _am fun._

15. I get mad when _I don't do well in school._

16. My mother never _lets me do stuff with friends._

17. I wish my father _would be home more._

18. I just can't _wait until I can start to drive and do more._

19. I'm different because _I stutter._

20. My best friend _likes to hang out with me._

Appropriate for ages 9 years and older

CLINICIAN'S COMMENTS

Several of **Caryn's** responses relate to stuttering. Her answers indicate strong negative beliefs and feelings about her stuttering problem, and that she has significant fears/worries associated with her speech. She does state however, that she talks a lot in school.

Paper-Pencil Task #8:
Count Me Out

DESCRIPTION/PURPOSE:

This task asks children to rank avoidance of selected speaking situations using always, sometimes, or never.

WHEN & HOW TO USE:

It is used most often with older children who report or are observed to exhibit avoidance of talking because of stuttering.

SPECIAL INSTRUCTIONS/NOTES:

This instrument is best administered orally so further probing can be used if necessary.

AN ALTERNATIVE PAPER-PENCIL TASK:

None.

Name:_____
Date:_____
Age:_____

"COUNT ME OUT"

Many people may avoid speaking in situations because they think they may stutter.

Read each statement below.
Check whether you would *Always, Sometimes* or *Never* avoid the situation.

	Always	*Sometimes*	*Never*
☐ Ordering for myself in a restaurant			
☐ Talking with friends			
☐ Asking for a date			
☐ Calling a store for information			
☐ Talking to an authority figure			
☐ Giving directions			
☐ Talking to my parents			
☐ Talking to a store clerk			
☐ Answering/talking on the phone			
☐ Giving a speech in class			
☐ Reading aloud			

Appropriate for ages 12 years and older

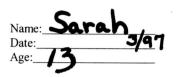

Name: **Sarah**
Date: **3/97**
Age: **13**

"COUNT ME OUT"

Many people may avoid speaking in situations because they think they may stutter.

Read each statement below.
Check whether you would *Always, Sometimes* or *Never* avoid the situation.

	Always	Sometimes	Never
☐ Ordering for myself in a restaurant		X	
☐ Talking with friends			X
☐ Asking for a date	wouldn't do it ☺		
☐ Calling a store for information			X
☐ Talking to an authority figure		X	
☐ Giving directions			X
☐ Talking to my parents			X
☐ Talking to a store clerk			X
☐ Answering/talking on the phone			X
☐ Giving a speech in class		X	
☐ Reading aloud		X	

Appropriate for ages 12 years and older

CLINICIAN'S COMMENTS

Sarah's responses showed the speaking situations she would "sometimes" avoid. This information assisted us in developing hierarchies (i.e., a series of steps from easiest to most difficult) later in therapy.

Paper-Pencil Task #9:
Worry Ladder

DESCRIPTION/PURPOSE:

The purpose of this instrument is to have the child list any worries they may have in rank order. This helps explore or discover a child's anxieties.

WHEN & HOW TO USE:

This task is best completed individually. Note whether communication problems are indicated and where they are ranked on the ladder.

SPECIAL INSTRUCTIONS/NOTES:

This task may also be used to have the child build a hierarchy of feared speaking situations.

AN ALTERNATIVE PAPER-PENCIL TASK:

None.

Name:_____

Date:_____

Age:_____

Worry Ladder

most

Write the things
you worry about
from the least to
the most

least

Appropriate for ages 9 years and older

Name: Pat

Date: 7/16

Age: 12

Worry Ladder

most

Write the things you worry about from the least to the most

Shots at the doctor ← (nobody likes shots)

Speaking in front of the school

Getting good grades

Going to the dentist

Having to make a long speech

Performing well in sports

Getting in Trouble

least

Appropriate for ages 9 years and older

CLINICIAN'S COMMENTS

Pat's ladder indicates specific concerns about communication in front of others. This ladder was completed during the assessment process.

Name: Danny
Date: 11/7
Age: 11

Worry Ladder

Write the things you worry about from the least to the most

most

Stuttering in front of school

Do a report out loud

Getting hert by anotha person

Talking to a person I don't know

Stuttering on PHONe

calling people

asking Questions in classroom

Talking to my friends

Stutter on Perpous

least

"Speech Worries"

Appropriate for ages 9 years and older

CLINICIAN'S COMMENTS

Danny's ladder, completed during therapy, was intended to create a hierarchy of speaking situations he feared. His responses suggest that he feels more comfortable stuttering in a familiar pattern or with familiar listeners rather than when speaking to someone unfamiliar or to a large audience.

Paper-Pencil Task #10:
Framing My Speech

DESCRIPTION/PURPOSE:

This task provides a list of vocabulary words used to label emotions, and asks the child to choose those which describe his feelings about stuttering.

WHEN & HOW TO USE:

This task is used with children who show direct awareness about stuttering.

SPECIAL INSTRUCTIONS/NOTES:

As with previous tasks, note positive versus negative words used to describe the stuttering problem. Children may think of their own words to describe their feelings.

AN ALTERNATIVE PAPER-PENCIL TASK:

None.

Name: _____

Date: _____

Age: _____

Framing My Speech

Choose words from the bottom
of the page that describe
how you feel about your stuttering.
Write them inside of the frame.

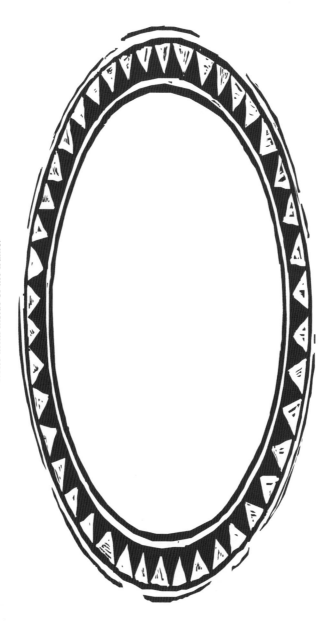

sad**happy**mixed-up**tired**frustrated**surprised**bad**hopeful**mad**bored**worried**smart**ashamed**lonely**disgusted**calm**shy**different**upset**relaxed**disappointed**brave**irritated**anxious**curious**pleased**weird**excited**afraid**confused**courageous**panicky**depressed**angry**embarrassed**annoyed**tense**guilty**proud**other**

Appropriate for ages 10 years and older

Name: Amanda
Date: 1/24
Age: 10 yrs

Framing My Speech

Choose words from the bottom
of the page that describe
how you feel about your stuttering.
Write them inside of the frame.

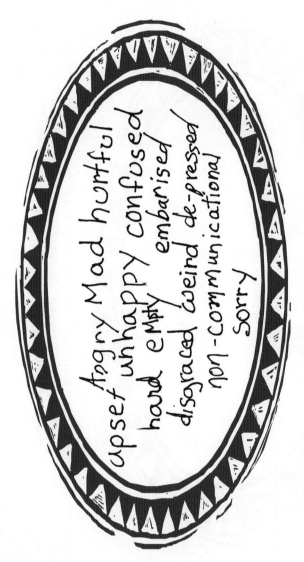

Angry Mad hurtful
upset unhappy confused
hard empty embarised
disgraced weind de-pressed
non-communication
Sorry

Appropriate for ages 10 years and older

sad**happy**mixed-up**tired**frustrated**surprised**bad**hopeful**mad**bored**worried**smart**ashamed*
lonely**disgusted**calm**shy**different**upset**relaxed**disappointed**brave**irritated**anxious**curious**
pleased**weird**excited**afraid**confused**courageous**panicky**depressed**angry**embarrassed**annoyed*
tense**guilty**proud**other**

CLINICIAN'S COMMENTS

All of **Amanda's** descriptors are negative. She included some words that were not part of the
original vocabulary set, such as "sorry," "disgraced," and "non-communicational."

Name: Robert
Date: 10-19
Age: 11

Framing My Speech

Choose words from the bottom
of the page that describe
how you feel about your stuttering.
Write them inside of the frame.

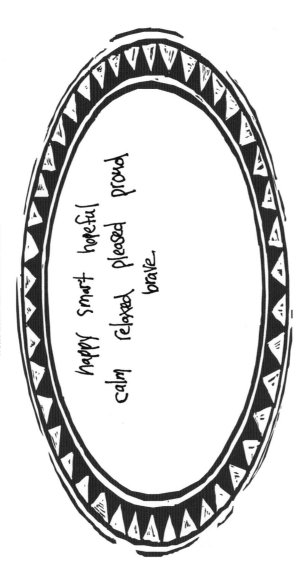

happy smart hopeful
calm relaxed pleased proud
brave

sad**happy**mixed-up**tired**frustrated**surprised**bad**hopeful**mad**bored**worried**smart**ashamed*
lonely**disgusted**calm**shy**different**upset**relaxed**disappointed**brave**irritated**anxious**curious**
pleased**weird**excited**afraid**confused**courageous**panicky**depressed**angry**embarrassed**annoyed**
tense**guilty**proud**other**

Appropriate for ages 10 years and older

CLINICIAN'S COMMENTS

Robert chose words indicating positive feelings about his stuttering.

66

Paper-Pencil Task #11:
Draw Me a Picture

DESCRIPTION/PURPOSE:

This self-portrait task provides insight into the child's emotions regarding his communication on days when talking is easy and days when it is more difficult.

WHEN & HOW TO USE:

This task can be used with children who show limited awareness of their stuttering or who demonstrate frustration with communication but have not yet directly mentioned stuttering. Ask the child to draw a picture of himself on a day when talking is easy and on a day when talking is "not so easy," "hard," or "difficult."

SPECIAL INSTRUCTIONS/NOTES:

If the child is reluctant to draw because of a lack of confidence in their artistic skills, it can be reassuring if you also draw a self-portrait. Pay particular attention to the expressions on the child's faces in the two separate drawings. Also, note how long it takes the child to complete each drawing. You might want to also ask the child why he/she included certain elements or facial expressions.

AN ALTERNATIVE PAPER-PENCIL TASK:

None.

Name: _____

Date: _____

Age: _____

What does your face look like on a talking day? _____

What does your face look like on a talking day? _____

Appropriate for ages five years and older

Name: Colby
Age: 5
Date: 10/11

What does your face look like on a
BUMPY _____ talking day?

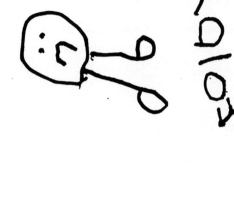

taloa

What does your face look like on a
EASY _____ talking day?

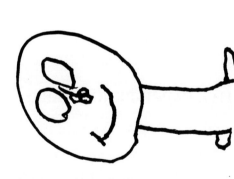

Appropriate for ages five years and older

C L I N I C I A N ' S   C O M M E N T S

Colby's mother had indicated that he was very self-conscious about his speech. When questioned, Colby told us he didn't worry about it. When we asked Colby to draw these pictures, however, we perceived some negative feelings about his stuttering.

Paper-Pencil Task #12:
My Family and I

DESCRIPTION/PURPOSE:

This drawing task can be used with younger or older children to elicit information about family communication patterns.

WHEN & HOW TO USE:

The child is asked to draw a picture of his family talking at the dinner table.

SPECIAL INSTRUCTIONS/NOTES:

It is interesting to note who is included in the picture, where they are, and what they are doing. Write down the child's interpretation of the picture when it is finished.

AN ALTERNATIVE PAPER-PENCIL TASK:

None.

Name:

Date:

Draw me a picture of.........................

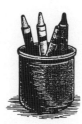

Who: your family
What: talking
Where: at the dinner table

Appropriate for ages 6 years and older

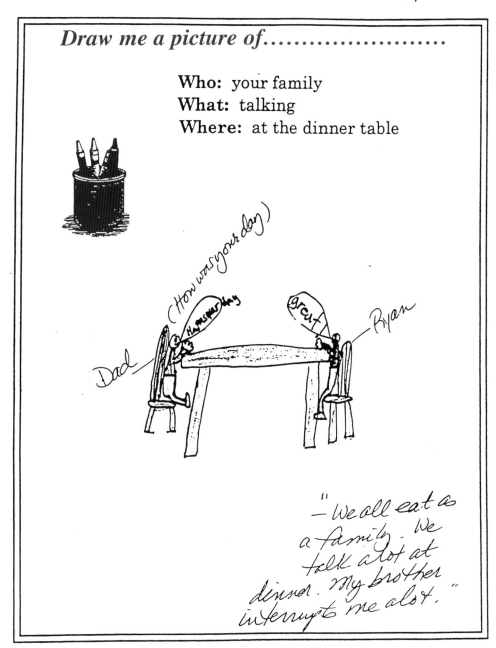

Draw me a picture of.........................

Who: your family
What: talking
Where: at the dinner table

Dad

(How was your day)

Happy day

great

Ryan

"— We all eat as a family. We talk a lot at dinner. My brother interrupts me alot."

Appropriate for ages 6 years and older

CLINICIAN'S COMMENTS

Ryan's drawing showed him talking with his dad at the dinner table. Although he stated that his whole family ate together, only Ryan and his father were in the picture. Ryan shared that his brother frequently interrupted him.

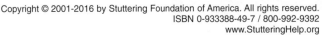

Paper-Pencil Task #13:
How Do I See My Stuttering?

DESCRIPTION/PURPOSE:

This task prompts the child to draw a picture that represents how he feels about stuttering. It provides a creative means for the child to express himself. The drawing may demonstrate a range of emotions about stuttering.

WHEN & HOW TO USE:

The child completes this task independently and then explains what the picture means. It is usually used for older children who can understand the task.

SPECIAL INSTRUCTIONS/NOTES:

None.

AN ALTERNATIVE PAPER-PENCIL TASK:

None.

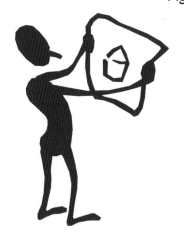

How do I "see" my stuttering?

Draw a picture on the back of this paper that shows how you feel about your stuttering problem. Write down what your picture means.

Appropriate for ages 9 years and older

Michael age 13

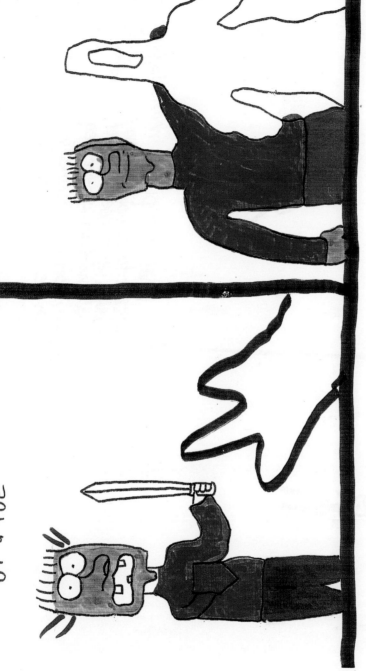

Stuttering can be a friend
or a foe

Although fighting it off does come around, if you work

hard enough at it, it doesn't seem to be as scary anymore.
It might turn to be a friend rather than a foe.
If you find it being a friend, talking gets easier.

age: 8
Sherese

Black dimond

inter mediate

What this picture means is one skier is
suppose to be going down a black diamond with
moguls, which means that sometimes my speech is
rough and too fast for people to understand.
Another skier is on an intermediate hill which means
my speech can be clear and I can use my tools.

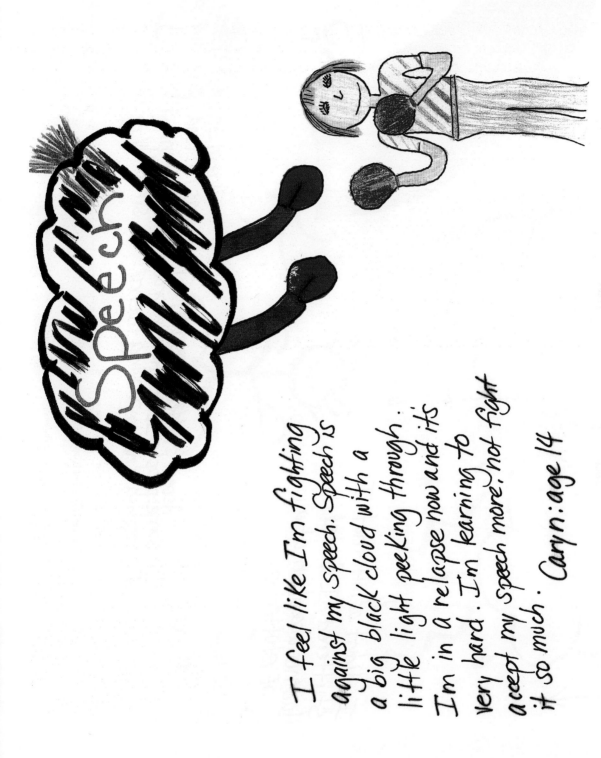

I feel like I'm fighting against my speech. Speech is a big black cloud with a little light peeking through. I'm in a relapse now and it's very hard. I'm learning to accept my speech more, not fight it so much. Caryn: age 14

CLINICIAN'S COMMENTS

Caryn's picture represents negative feelings she experienced during a period of relapse.

Copyright © 2001-2016 by Stuttering Foundation of America. All rights reserved.
ISBN 0-933388-49-7 / 800-992-9392
www.StutteringHelp.org

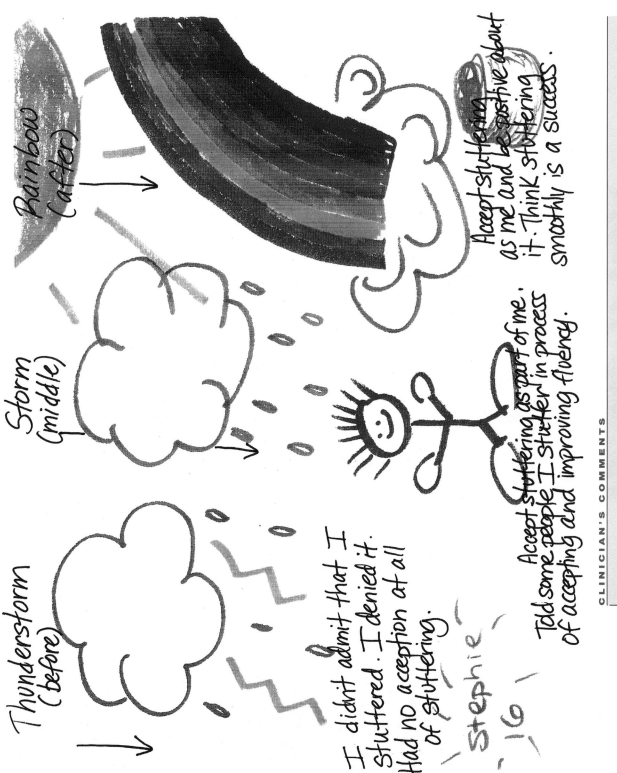

Rainbow (after)

Storm (middle)

Thunderstorm (before)

I didn't admit that I stuttered. I denied it. Had no acception at all of stuttering.

Accept stuttering as part of me. Told some people I stutter in process of accepting and improving fluency.

Accept stuttering as me and be positive about it. Think stuttering smoothly is a success.

Stephie 16

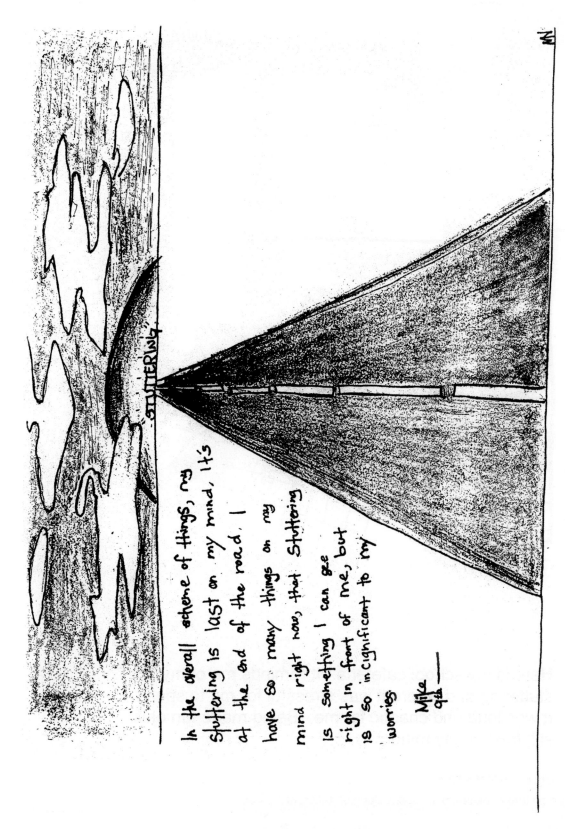

In the overall scheme of things, my stuttering is last on my mind. It's at the end of the road. I have so many things on my mind right now, that stuttering is something I can get right in front of me, but is so insignificant to my worries

Mike
9th

Landon
age 15 grade 10

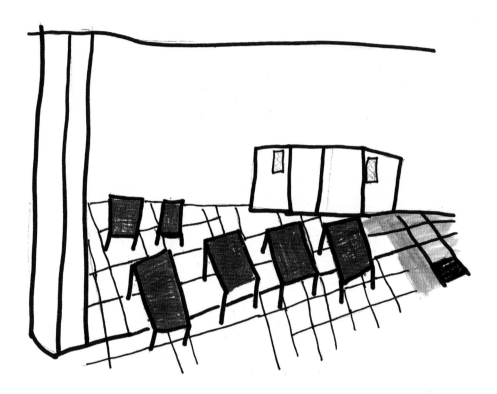

Here is my school cafeteria. It reminds me of my
stuttering and where it was stressful for me to speak.
It was loud and chaotic for me. Being made fun of is
still fresh in my mind.

CLINICIAN'S COMMENTS

Landon's picture depicts a difficult speaking situation at school.

Brad   Age 10

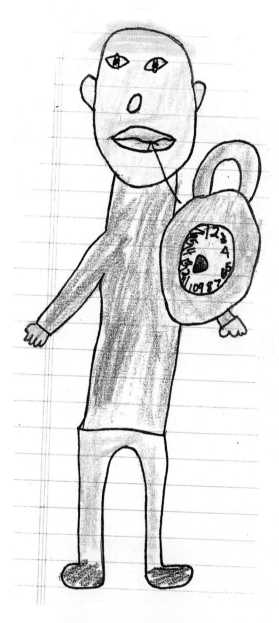

My lips are locked up. I'm stuttering. The lock has a combination to open it. And the combination is to use tools and practice.

CLINICIAN'S COMMENTS

Brad's picture describes his stuttering and his understanding that speech tools can make talking easier.

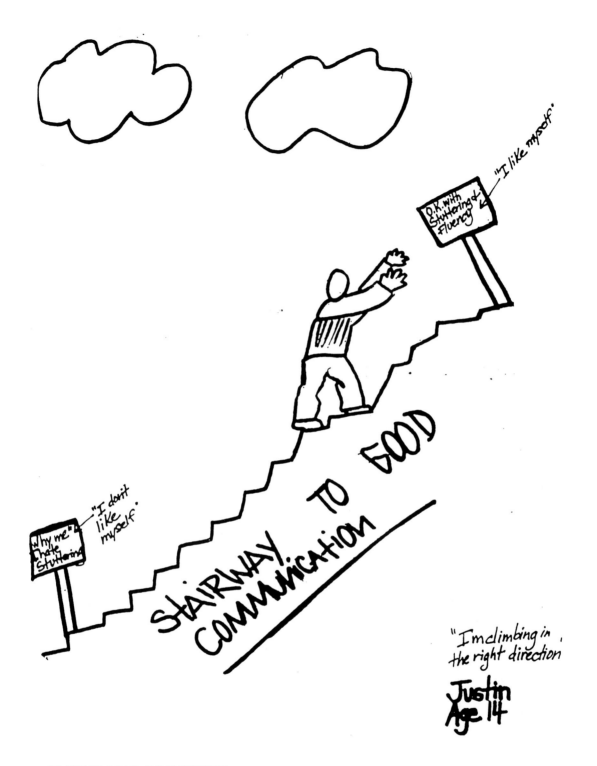

Paper-Pencil Task #14:
Parent Questionnaire

DESCRIPTION/PURPOSE:

This task includes 10 open-ended statements to obtain parents' perceptions about the stuttering problem.

WHEN & HOW TO USE IT:

This task is used as part of the case history during the evaluation process.

SPECIAL INSTRUCTIONS/NOTES:

Each parent completes his or her own questionnaire. This allows us to further understand both perceptions.

AN ALTERNATIVE PAPER-PENCIL TASK:

None.

Teacher Questionnaire

Name of Child: _____

Teacher: _____

Grade/Section: _____

Date: _____

Return form to: _____

Please complete the following statements:

1. Some things I have noticed about this child's communication are...

2. When this child answers questions in class, he/she...

3. When this child speaks to me at my desk, he/she...

4. When this child reads aloud, he/she...

5. If/When this child has difficulty speaking, I respond by...

6. If/When this child has difficulty speaking, other children respond by...

7. If/When this child has difficulty speaking, it occurs mostly when...

8. My knowledge about stuttering is...

9. Other concerns I have about this child's success in the classroom are...

10. Most importantly, right now I need to know...

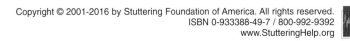

Paper-Pencil Task #14:
Parent Questionnaire

DESCRIPTION/PURPOSE:

This task includes 10 open-ended statements to obtain parents' perceptions about the stuttering problem.

WHEN & HOW TO USE IT:

This task is used as part of the case history during the evaluation process.

SPECIAL INSTRUCTIONS/NOTES:

Each parent completes his or her own questionnaire. This allows us to further understand both perceptions.

AN ALTERNATIVE PAPER-PENCIL TASK:

None.

Parent Questionnaire

Name of Child: _____

Name of Parent(s): _____

Date: _____

Please complete the following statements:

1. My greatest concerns regarding my child's speech problem are...

2. I feel my child is/is not aware of his/her speech problem because...

3. I feel my child is/is not concerned about his/her speech problem because...

4. The situations where my child has the most trouble talking are...

5. When my child stutters, I feel...

6. When my child stutters, I say/do...

7. When my child stutters, other family members react by...

8. My knowledge about stuttering is...

9. From previous therapy, if any, I learned...

10. As a result of this therapy, I hope...

Paper-Pencil Task #15:
Teacher Questionnaire

DESCRIPTION/PURPOSE:

This task includes 10 open-ended statements to obtain teachers' perceptions about the stuttering problem.

WHEN & HOW TO USE IT:

This task is used as part of the case history during the evaluation process.

SPECIAL INSTRUCTIONS/NOTES:

If the child has more than one teacher, have each fill out their own copy.

AN ALTERNATIVE PAPER-PENCIL TASK:

None.

Teacher Questionnaire

Name of Child: _____

Teacher: _____

Grade/Section: _____

Date: _____

Return form to: _____

Please complete the following statements:

1. Some things I have noticed about this child's communication are…

2. When this child answers questions in class, he/she…

3. When this child speaks to me at my desk, he/she…

4. When this child reads aloud, he/she…

5. If/When this child has difficulty speaking, I respond by…

6. If/When this child has difficulty speaking, other children respond by…

7. If/When this child has difficulty speaking, it occurs mostly when…

8. My knowledge about stuttering is…

9. Other concerns I have about this child's success in the classroom are…

10. Most importantly, right now I need to know…

Chapter 4

treatment

Specific treatment strategies can be used to help children develop or maintain positive attitudes and feelings. Certainly, changes in speech behaviors are also an important component of therapy, although they will not be covered in this book. If you need more information on developing goals and objectives for changes in speech behavior as well as strategies for achieving these types of changes, please refer to the references at the end of this book.

As previously stated, each child who stutters has unique needs. Therefore some strategies presented in this chapter may not be appropriate for every child.

The information you have from the assessment will help you develop appropriate goals as well as highlight ways you will document progress over time. Before writing a goal for a child, we ask the following questions:

➤ What evidence do you have that such a goal is necessary?

➤ How will you show progress in measurable ways?

➤ What strategies will be necessary, and how will you implement them in a way that matches the child's age, cognitive ability, and awareness of the problem?

The long-term goal for this aspect of therapy is straightforward: the child will either *develop* or *maintain* positive attitudes and feelings about stuttering, communication, and self.

For example, Johnny, age 10, exhibited negative attitudes and feelings and reported little knowledge about stuttering. He was demonstrating avoidance of stuttering and little oral participation in the classroom. He believed that he could stop stuttering if he just tried hard enough. Therefore, Johnny's long-term goal was to *develop* positive attitudes and feelings about stuttering, communication, and self, by increasing his knowledge about stuttering, decreasing avoidance, and increasing classroom participation.

On the other hand, Tess, age 8, stuttered freely in the home and school environments. While she was aware of the problem, she reported that it didn't bother her and the observations we made during the assessment process supported her statements. As a result, her long-term goal for this component of therapy was to *maintain* positive attitudes and feelings about stuttering, communication, and self by increasing her understanding of the problem, continuing to be open about her stuttering, and not avoiding it.

Utilizing a variety of concrete strategies helps us either develop or maintain positive attitudes and feelings. Some children may view stuttering as something bad, scary, or as something that they shouldn't be doing.

Providing information, such as learning about talking and stuttering, assists children in understanding what's happening when speech breakdowns occur. This information is just as important for children who are *not* experiencing negative attitudes and feelings as for those who *are*. Demystifying stuttering may help them learn to change the way they think and feel about the problem (Murphy, 1996). Ultimately this results in changes in how they learn to cope with it.

It is also important to provide ways for children to identify issues related to their stuttering, and to develop skills for independent problem-solving. Some children need to learn that the ways they talk to themselves about the problem can influence how they feel. They also need to learn that the way we think about this problem can be changed.

Many children also experience fears associated with communication, either of stuttering itself or of speaking in certain environments. Learning new ways of accepting stuttering more openly and working through speaking fears are important. In doing so, they can learn to manage more effectively.

As we discuss specific strategies, notice that some directly involve parents and teachers. By increasing their understanding of stuttering, the child's experience, and the treatment process, you will facilitate progress in therapy.

Parents and teachers can also learn new ways of understanding and talking with the child about the problem. In our experience, children change attitudes about stuttering as others around them talk about it in similar ways. When families and teachers are involved in treatment, children can learn to use these skills in the home and classroom environments.

The following strategies may be used when working to develop or maintain positive attitudes and feelings. They represent concrete, measurable ways to assist children in achieving attitudinal change. Because stuttering and associated attitudes and feelings are constantly changing and are different for each child, the challenge lies in selecting and implementing appropriate strategies to meet the child's needs at any given time in therapy.

For each described strategy, we will include (1) its purpose, (2) special considerations for use, and (3) possible short-term objectives, followed by clinical examples. The strategies are not necessarily used in the exact sequence presented, but rather introduced to each child in a sequence that is based on his or her individual needs. We must remember, however, that the way we relate to the child creates the foundation for making affective and cognitive changes.

Strategy 1: Creating a Speech Notebook

DESCRIPTION/PURPOSE:

The speech notebook is a documentation tool that provides a concrete means for children to understand issues about stuttering and speech therapy in an ongoing manner. Most importantly, it creates a non-verbal medium for expressing feelings and for understanding the connection between thinking, feeling, and talking. It is an important tool for referring back to previous therapy activities, understanding variability of the problem, and for noting progress. It helps the child teach parents and others about stuttering and stuttering therapy.

INSTRUCTIONS FOR USE:

The speech notebook is created at the beginning of therapy, and we've found a 3-ring binder works best. On a regular basis, copies of the notebook pages should be made and kept in the child's file to document and illustrate progress. The child uses the speech notebook as an archive of what is accomplished in therapy.

SHORT-TERM OBJECTIVE:

The child will create and maintain a speech notebook for use in therapy sessions throughout the academic year.

Strategy 2: Learning About Talking and Stuttering

DESCRIPTION/PURPOSE:

Learning about talking and stuttering helps the child develop an understanding of what happens when he or she stutters. It also lays the foundation for learning specific tools to make talking easier. Three concepts are emphasized: (1) the body parts involved in creating speech; (2) the process or order by which speech happens; and, (3) the choices we have when producing speech. This activity helps children understand *why* they stutter (i.e., "sometimes our speech machine doesn't work the way we want it to"), what they are *doing* when talking becomes harder, and that there are *choices* they can make about making it easier. Learning about talking in this way (i.e., "I understand, I know, and I have choices") prepares the foundation as the clinician and child negotiate what will help make it easier. This is an important attitude and helps motivate children to change.

INSTRUCTIONS FOR USE:

Analogies are a good way to implement this strategy. For example, we have used Ramig and Bennett's (1995) speech pizza activity. This activity includes asking the child to list *ingredients* needed for a basic pizza, then discussing and drawing the *order* in which these ingredients are put together to make a pizza. Finally, brainstorming and listing all *choices* for toppings is followed by a discussion of the child's favorite choices. Making a real pizza is a memorable activity the following session! The pizza-making activity "sets the stage" for talking about how we make talking.

The child is then asked, "What do you think we need to make talking?" Body *parts* are listed (often with our assistance) in the speech notebook and include the diaphragm, lungs, voice box, vocal cords,

91

mouth, lips, tongue, teeth, and brain. Next the child's torso is traced on chart paper or sketched in the speech notebook and all body parts are drawn in, colored, and labeled. Then we discuss *how talking happens* and brainstorm *choices* that every speaker has (e.g., loud, soft, high, low, bumpy, smooth, etc.). We consistently refer back to this diagram throughout therapy. Learning about talking makes talking about stuttering more objective. It can decrease sensitivity about the problem as the child becomes more objective about it.

If appropriate, some children benefit from learning more about stuttering. Definitions, how people stutter, and theories of stuttering can be listed in the notebook. Facts and myths about stuttering and famous people who stutter can also be included.

SHORT-TERM OBJECTIVE:

The child will diagram and discuss the process of speech production.

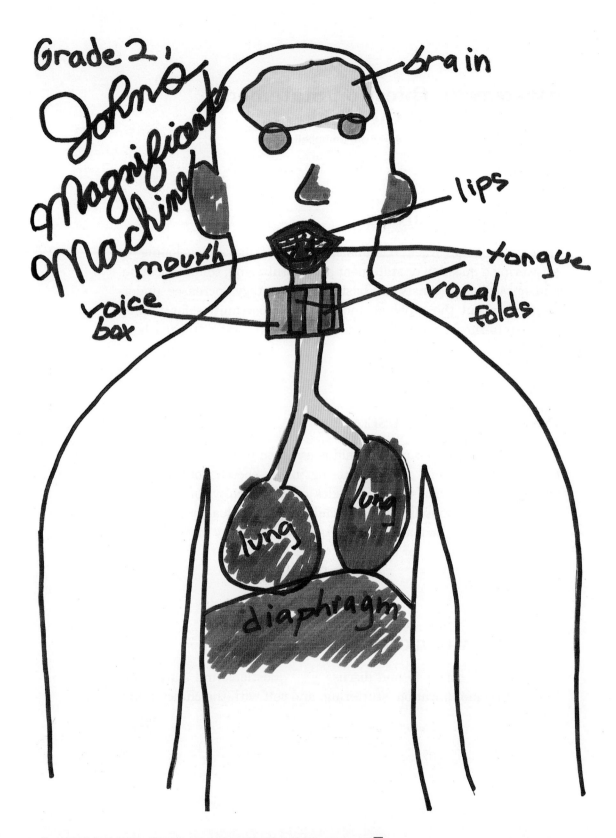

Grade 2,
John's
Magnificiant
Machine

brain

lips

tongue

mouth

vocal folds

voice box

lung

lung

diaphragm

Strategy 3: Question/Statement of the Week
(adapted from Campbell, 1998)

DESCRIPTION/PURPOSE:

Question of the Week (Campbell, 1998) includes developing or answering a question or statement about stuttering, communication, and oneself on a consistent basis. This strategy increases understanding about the problem and creates opportunities for talking about stuttering between the child, us, the parents, and/or the teachers.

INSTRUCTIONS FOR USE:

From the onset of therapy, the child is assigned to write a question or complete a statement about stuttering in the speech notebook on a weekly (or other) basis. This provides an opportunity for discussion based on the information given. The child may also ask a question of the clinician, parents, or teachers in the notebook, or they may present a question or statement for the child.

SHORT-TERM OBJECTIVE:

The child will complete and discuss ____ questions and statements related to communication, stuttering, and self with the clinician and others.

Questions to ask Cate:
Age 10

Miss Kristin :

- What was the Hardest thing about starting?

- Did people disrespet you?

- When did friends liking you for who you are?

Strategy 4: Meaningful Topics for Discussion

DESCRIPTION/PURPOSE:

Meaningful Topics for Discussion assists the child in identifying and understanding issues related to progress in therapy. It also helps us highlight, explore, and teach children how these topics relate to stuttering. This strategy is helpful when discussing abstract concepts such as responsibility, motivation, change, etc.

INSTRUCTIONS FOR USE:

Three methods we use to identify and explore Meaningful Topics for Discussion are: (1) webbing or concept mapping, (2) flow charts, and (3) rating scales.

Webbing/Concept Mapping: A concept or issue is identified based on something we see the child do or something we hear the child say. A specific word is often used to represent the issue and questions are generated relating to its definition, its importance in real life, and its connection to stuttering. A concept map may also be developed to explore a specific issue.

Flow charts: Flow charts are used most often to illustrate how a chain of events can ultimately affect one another. They may include stick figures or pictures of key elements. Most often, they are used to illustrate the relationships between thinking, feeling, and talking.

Rating scale: These are best used to show changes over time, including variability and progress. You may ask a child to make a rating in several different ways: on a numerical scale (e.g., one to five), on a word scale (e.g., best to worst), or on a pictorial scale (e.g., with faces showing different levels of emotion). Examples may include rating how much talking bothers a child, how much a child feels he's learned about the problem, or how afraid a child is about speaking in class.

SHORT-TERM OBJECTIVE:

The child will document and explain ___ issues related to the stuttering problem with clinician and others.

Amy age 12

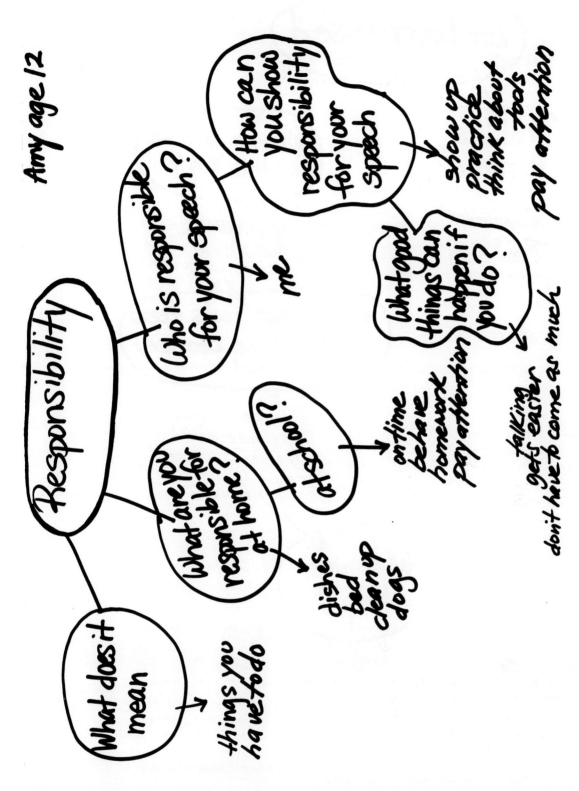

Responsibility

What does it mean → things you have to do

What are you responsible for at home? → dishes, bad, cleanup dogs

at school? → on time, behave, homework, pay attention

Who is responsible for your speech? → me

How can you show responsibility for your speech → show up, practice, think about tools, pay attention

What good things can happen if you do? → talking gets easier, don't have to come as much

CLINICIAN'S COMMENTS

Amy, age 12, had frequent absences from therapy and was not completing home assignments. We used a web to address the issue of "responsibility" as a meaningful topic for discussion.

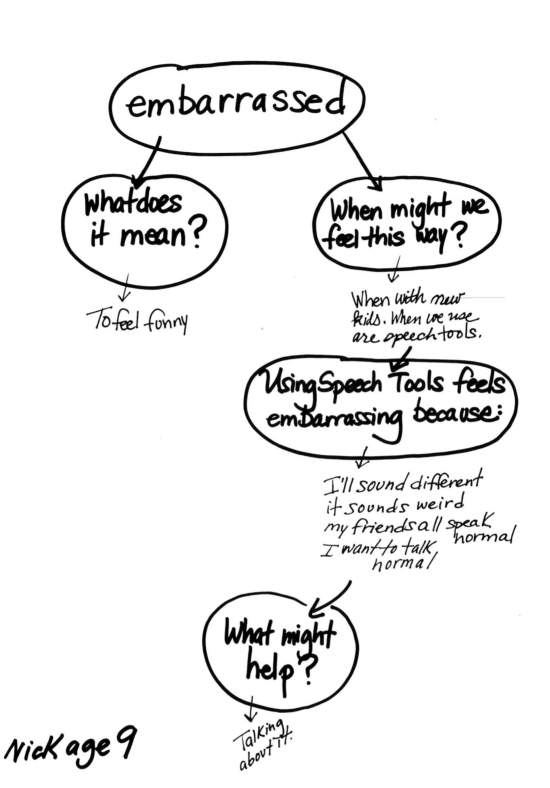

embarrassed

What does it mean?

→ To feel funny

When might we feel this way?

When with new kids. When we use are speech tools.

Using Speech Tools feels embarrassing because:

I'll sound different
it sounds weird
my friends all speak normal
I want to talk normal

What might help?

→ Talking about it.

Nick age 9

CLINICIAN'S COMMENTS

Nick's mother shared that he wouldn't use speech tools at school because he was embarrassed. This was then discussed using a web.

Frank
age 12

Relapse

1. What does it mean?
If something is doing good than it gets bad changes.

2. What does it have to do with life?
When someones is sick

3. What does it have to do with stuttering?
It's just part of the problem (Relapse)

4. Name 5 reasons why it's a great thing?
1. Gets us to pay attention.
2. Provides opportunity for change.
3. It helps us talk about stuttering.
4. It helps us learn to manage better.
5. Gives opportunity to improve on tools.

CLINICIAN'S COMMENTS

Frank returned to therapy and asked, "Why has my talking gotten bad again?" The concept of relapse was discussed and a flow chart was created to help Frank understand the relationship between his thoughts, feelings and stuttering.

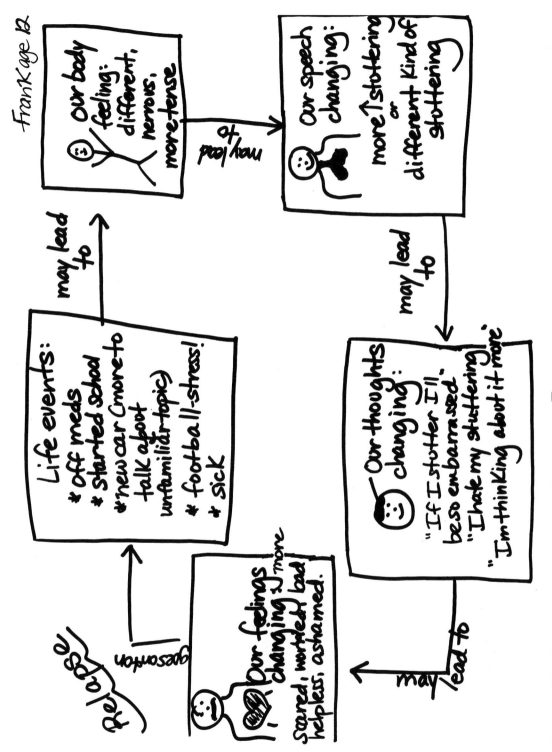

Frank age 12

Our body feeling: different, nervous, more tense

may lead to

Our speech changing: more ↑ stuttering or different kind of stuttering

may lead to

Our thoughts changing: "If I stutter I'll be so embarrassed." "I hate my stuttering." "I'm thinking about it more."

may lead to

Our feelings changing: ↑ more scared, worried, bad, helpless, ashamed.

prevention

Relapse

Life events:
* off meds
* started school
* new car (more to talk about - unfamiliar topic)
* football - stress!
* sick

may lead to

Matthew age:6

When talking gets
bumpy

I stop +
I wait +
I start over easy

And my
talking comes
out smooth

CLINICIAN'S COMMENTS

Matthew's flow chart illustrates his understanding of using speech tools.

Umang 12 yrs.

Paying attention

What does it mean?
Know what you are doing + think about it. Focus on a certain something

What kinds of things do you usually have to pay attention to?
Something new you are just being taught. School, sports

↓

School lectures, School homework, during game in Sports, class disussions

Why do you have to pay attention during the game in sports?
If you don't, you won't know what to do when you get the ball or something & you might get hurt if not

What about talking do you have to pay attention to?
How it feels What you say, how you say it, Tension

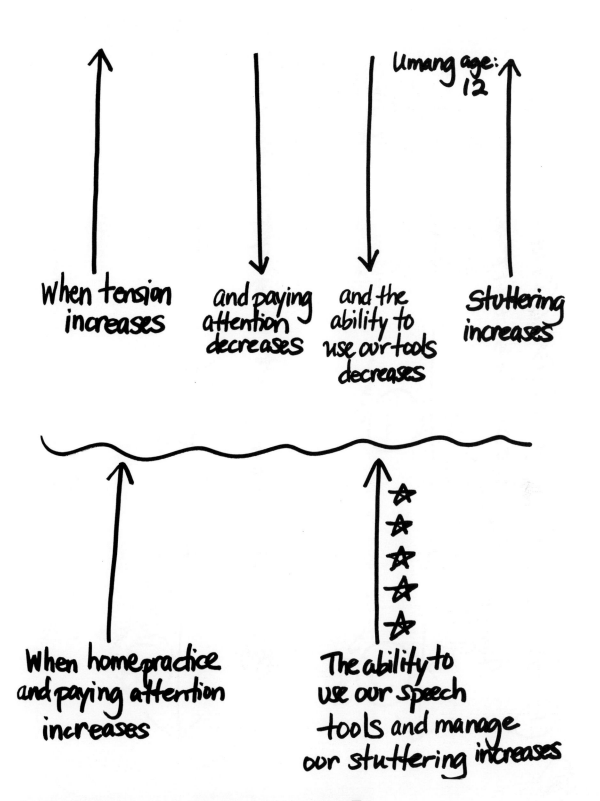

When tension increases

and paying attention decreases

and the ability to use our tools decreases

Umang age: 12

Stuttering increases

When home practice and paying attention increases

The ability to use our speech tools and manage our stuttering increases

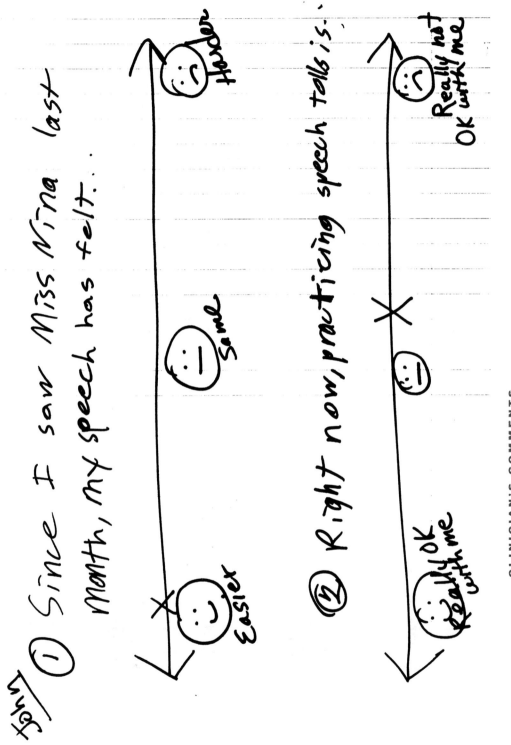

John ①

Since I saw Miss Nina last month, my speech has felt...

Harder

☺

Same

☺

Easier

② Right now, practicing speech talk is...

Really not OK with me

☺

Really OK with me

☺

CLINICIAN'S COMMENTS

John's rating scale illustrates his monitoring of how speech has felt over time and his feelings about home practice.

Copyright © 2001-2016 by Stuttering Foundation of America. All rights reserved.
ISBN 0-933388-49-7 / 800-992-9392
www.StutteringHelp.org

104

Justin 13

① How much does my speech bug me?

|————————————✗—7
Not   very
at all   much!

② How much do I like the way I talk?

|✗————————————7
I don't   I like it fine
like it.
I hate it

③ How much do I want to change the way I talk?

|————————————✗—7
I really want to   It doesn't really
change   matter.

CLINICIAN'S COMMENTS

Justin's rating scale illustrates his dislike for stuttering and possible lack of motivation for making further speech changes.

Copyright © 2001-2016 by Stuttering Foundation of America. All rights reserved.
ISBN 0-933388-49-7 / 800-992-9392
www.StutteringHelp.org

Strategy 5: Problem-Solving Plan

DESCRIPTION/PURPOSE:

The Problem-Solving Plan is a series of steps used by the child to identify, create, and choose appropriate solutions for solving problems. It teaches the child to deal with present and future challenges related not only to stuttering but to life as well. The previous strategy, Meaningful Topics for Discussion, often creates opportunities to develop Problem-Solving Plans.

INSTRUCTIONS FOR USE:

A Problem-Solving Plan is documented in the Speech Notebook using the following steps:

1. Name the problem: "The problem is ..."

2. Fill in the blanks: "I feel ___ because ___ and I want ___."

3. Brainstorm possible solutions: "Say/write anything."
   All possible solutions are accepted without judgment in this step.

4. Discuss consequences of each choice: "If ____, then ___; choose one or more solutions."

5. Create a plan for follow-up.

SHORT-TERM OBJECTIVE:

The child will develop and explain ___ Problem-Solving Plans using the five step process.

The Problem is... my parents are coming up with their own ways to help my speech.

This makes me feel... Unhappy **because**... no one listens **and I want**... Them to just learn a little more about speech and how I feel

Brainstorm ideas : ① To come in for some more speech classes.

② To learn a new way of comunicating

③ To have my parents watch videos of speech when they cannot make it to lessons

④ have them ask me questions about my speech.

Discuss Consequences "If___, then___."

all are helpful ideas to help them learn to not tell me to "start over" or finish my sentences.

Choose 1 to try

I choose # 3 first.

Let's talk about your choice and how it worked on Jan. 23rd!!

Juanita – Age 10

CLINICIAN'S COMMENTS

This plan was created in response to **Juanita's** frustration regarding her parents' difficulty understanding her speech problem.

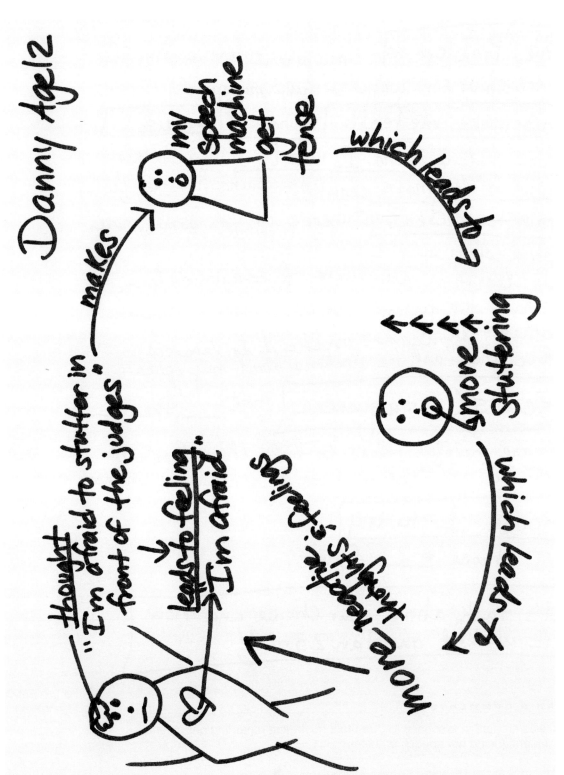

Danny Age12

my speech machine get tense

which leads to

makes

thought
"I'm afraid to stutter in
front of the judges"

leads to feeling
"I'm afraid"

more stuttering without speaking

which leads to

more
Stuttering

CLINICIAN'S COMMENTS

Before creating a problem-solving plan, a flow chart was made regarding **Danny**'s fear of talking in front of the judges at the science fair.

Problem Solving Plan

Danny
Age 12

1) **The problem is:** I am afraid of stuttering in front of the judges at the science fair.

2) I feel _afraid_ because _I might stutter_ and I want _to feel less afraid_ .

3) **Brainstorm Solutions:**
   — Admit to being afraid
   — Practice the speech with mom before the science fair.
   — Be open about stuttering with the judges. Tell them I stutter at the start.

   — use some tools.

4) **Discuss Consequences:**
   If I choose all of these, _then_ I will feel less afraid.

5) **Create Follow up Plan:** I'll do all and talk about it next week at speech.

CLINICIAN'S COMMENTS

A problem-solving plan was developed with **Danny.**

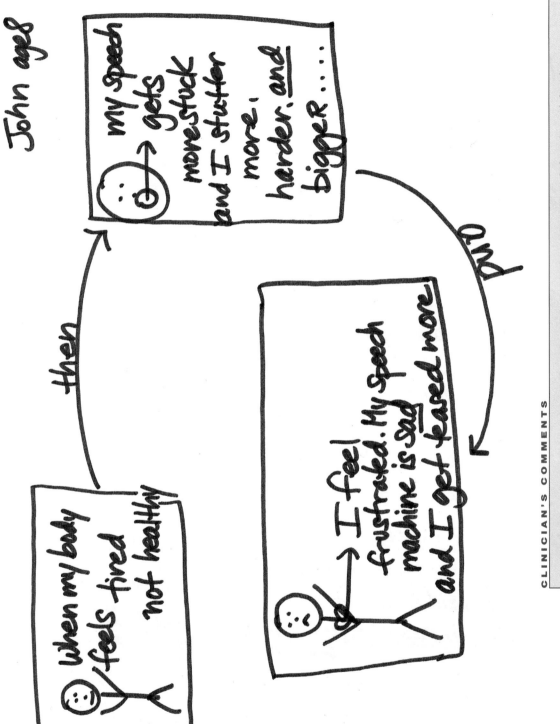

John age 8

when my body feels tired not healthy

then

my speech → gets more stuck and I stutter more, harder, and <u>bigger</u> . . . .

and

→ I feel frustrated. My speech machine is sad and I get teased more

CLINICIAN'S COMMENTS

Again, a flow chart was created before a problem-solving plan when **John** shared that he was having more trouble talking and was being teased by some neighbor boys.

Problem Solving Plan — John age 8

1. <u>The problem is</u> . . . . . My friends in my neighborhood are teasing me about my speech.

2. <u>I feel</u>: sad <u>because</u>: my friends are teasing <u>and I want</u>: them to stop.

3. <u>Possible Solutions</u>:

- walk away
- tell them "Don't Tease me"
- stare at them silently
- explain that I stutter sometimes
- ignore it
- tell someone
- talk about it with my mom and my friends

- ~~punch them~~
- ~~tease them back~~

together

4. <u>Consequences</u>: most were helpful, some were hurtful. From this (if...then) I chose

<u>If I tell them</u> "Don't tease me" they will stop.

5. <u>Follow-up plan</u>: Talk about it next week at speech

Reacting to the Teasing : Discussion

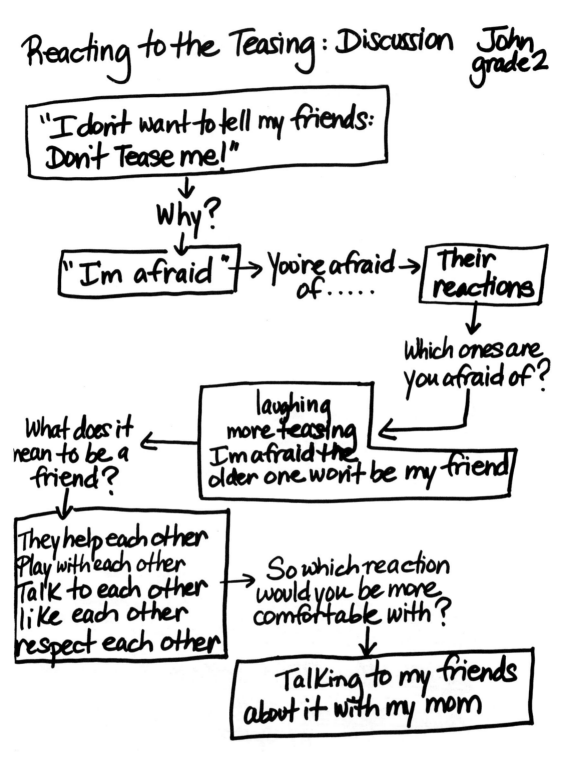

"I don't want to tell my friends: Don't Tease me!"

↓

Why?

↓

"I'm afraid" → You're afraid of..... → Their reactions

↓

Which ones are you afraid of?

laughing
more teasing
I'm afraid the older one won't be my friend

What does it mean to be a friend?

↓

They help each other
Play with each other
Talk to each other
like each other
respect each other

→ So which reaction would you be more comfortable with?

↓

Talking to my friends about it with my mom

CLINICIAN'S COMMENTS

The following week, **John** shared that he did not follow through with the plan and a flow chart was created to find out why.

112

10/18

① What is teasing?

Tim: When you make a joke about someone
Making fun of people.

Garret: When you make fun of someone

John: Making fun of someone or making a
joke about someone.

② How does it make someone
feel to be teased?

Garret: Makes someone feel bad.

Tim: Makes people feel sad

③ Do good friends tease
(in a hurtful way?)

Garret/Tim: No

④ What would be some ways to
react to John's speech?

Tim: I don't know.

Garret: Help him by saying the word

CLINICIAN'S COMMENTS

Following discussion about this flow chart, **John** decided to talk with his mom and the boys about his stuttering. His mother explored the concept of "teasing" and listed the boys' answers. This was returned to the clinician at the next therapy session.

113

10/20   John's ideas for friends →

Best ways to react when I am stuck:

① watch me with eye contact

② wait for me

③ give me my talking time

④ don't finish words for me

Strategy 6: Changing Our Thinking

DESCRIPTION/PURPOSE:

Changing Our Thinking is a strategy used to help children learn how to change negative thoughts into more positive ones. This helps children develop more positive attitudes about their stuttering and about themselves.

INSTRUCTIONS FOR USE:

Reframing: Initially, general negative thoughts are brainstormed, such as "I'm too fat," "I'm dumb in math," or "I'll never make the team." Negative thoughts about stuttering and communication are then listed. We use statements we've heard the child make in the past, and/or the child may share internal thoughts he has had. Then, we assist the child in changing the negative, or hurtful, thoughts into more positive, or helpful, ones. These negative thoughts are continuously "caught" and reframed throughout therapy (Ramig & Bennett, 1997).

Garbage Ball: This activity allows children the opportunity to brainstorm negative thoughts about themselves or an issue related to therapy and "get rid of them" in a concrete way. Specifically, we help the child write down negative thoughts about an issue. The paper is then rolled up into a ball, sealed with masking tape, and thrown away. Then, as "alternative" thoughts about the topic evolve, they are written down and reviewed periodically to show the child how his thoughts are changing.

SHORT-TERM OBJECTIVE:

The child will document negative thoughts and reframe them into more positive alternatives in ___ / ___ opportunities.

Negative Thoughts Kids might say to themselves:

Tim: age 10

I can't run fast enough.

I'm dumb in math.

I'm fat.

I'm not cool.

I look like a dork.

No one wants to be my friend.

Tim. age 10

Negative thoughts I have about stuttering →	Changing them to more positive ones
My speech is horrible.	I'm working on my speech.
I'm not good at speech tools.	My eye contact is getting better.
No one likes to hear me talk.	My friends are interested in my stories.
I hate my stuttering.	Stuttering is a tough problem to deal with.

CLINICIAN'S COMMENTS

Next, **Tim** listed four negative thoughts about his stuttering. We had heard these often during treatment. Then we helped Tim reframe or change those negative thoughts into more positive ones.

What I hate most about stuttering:

Scott
Age 14

It calls attention to me.

I hate how it feels.

I hate how I worry about ordering food.

I hate how unpredictable it is.

I hate how it makes me feel embarrassed.

I hate how I feel out of control.

I hate how it's hard to tell jokes.

I hate how people look at me.

I hate how I choose not to talk sometimes.

I even hate how much I hate my stuttering!

and
I hate how easy talking is for everyone else!!!

CLINICIAN'S COMMENTS

Scott demonstrated negative attitudes and feelings about his stuttering. We helped him list everything he hated about stuttering. The list became a garbage ball and was thrown away.

Strategy 7: The Speech Hierarchy

DESCRIPTION/PURPOSE:

A speech hierarchy is a series of identified steps towards achieving a specific goal. These steps are usually rank-ordered from easiest to hardest. A hierarchy used in this way helps children become desensitized to fears associated with speaking in certain situations.

Hierarchies are used in a similar fashion when teaching speech modification skills. Manipulating variables across the hierarchy (e.g., topic, model) helps the child achieve success at each step. This success helps build positive attitudes.

INSTRUCTIONS FOR USE:

We or the child may identify a difficult speaking situation. Other strategies, (e.g., webbing/concept mapping or flow charts) may be used to further explore the topic before a hierarchy is developed. Next, a series of small systematic steps are created from easiest to most difficult and listed on the hierarchy. Finally, the clinician helps the child work through each step in the hierarchy.

SHORT-TERM OBJECTIVE:

The child will identify ___ difficult speaking situations and develop and execute steps in the speech hierarchy.

Fear

↓

What does "fear" mean?

To be afraid, scared of something.

What kinds of things are people afraid of?

Mices, Rollercoasters, Guns

What kinds of things are you afraid of?

Failing in school, drugs, talking on the phone.

What kinds of things do people fear when they stutter?

Phone, speeches, girls

Do you have any situations that you are afraid of talking in? The phone

Is "fear" o.k. ??

No Yes

CLINICIAN'S COMMENTS

After identifying fear as a Meaningful Topic for Discussion, **Ben** was able to pinpoint talking on the phone as a feared speaking situation.

Ben: age 11
Part 2

When I think and feel "afraid" about talking / stuttering on the phone

my body (and my speech mechanism) gets TENSE!

and

Talking is even harder!

and

I feel more afraid next time!

CLINICIAN'S COMMENTS

A flowchart was created to help **Ben** understand the relationship between thoughts and feelings about "fear," body tension, and stuttering.

Ben - age 11
Part 2

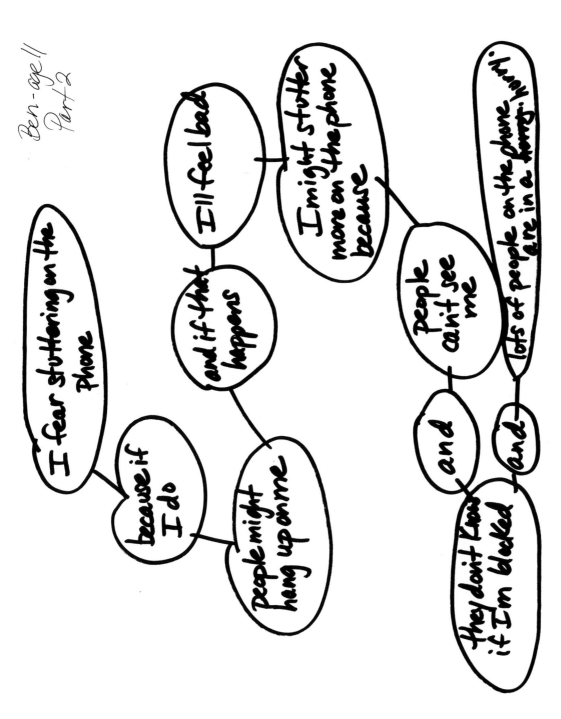

- I fear stuttering on the phone
- because if I do
- People might hang up on me
- and if that happens
- I'll feel bad
- I might stutter more on the phone because
- People can't see me
  - and
  - they don't know if I'm blocked
- and
- lots of people on the phone are in a hurry/wan't

CLINICIAN'S COMMENTS

Next, possible reasons why the phone was scary to **Ben** were brainstormed using a web.

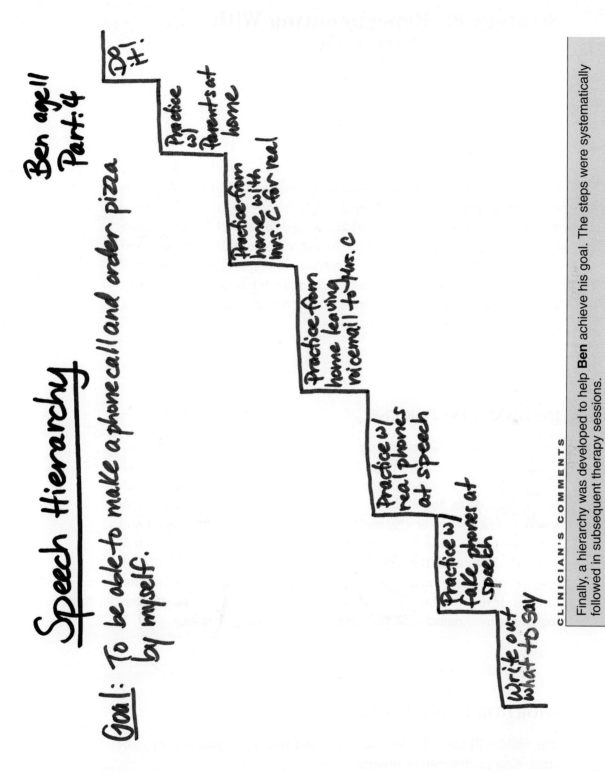

Speech Hierarchy

Ben age 11
Part 4

Goal: To be able to make a phone call and order pizza by myself.

Do it.

Practice (x) Parents at home

Practice from home with Mrs. C for real

Practice from home leaving voicemail to Mrs. C

Practice w/ real phones at speech

Practice w/ fake phones at speech

Write out what to say

CLINICIAN'S COMMENTS

Finally, a hierarchy was developed to help **Ben** achieve his goal. The steps were systematically followed in subsequent therapy sessions.

Strategy 8: Experimenting With Stuttering

DESCRIPTION/PURPOSE:

This strategy is used to desensitize children or make them more comfortable and less anxious about the moment of stuttering. This decrease in fear of the stuttering moment may result in decreased bodily tension, allowing the child to manage the speech problem more effectively (Murphy, 1996). This strategy helps children put their stuttering "out in the open." It serves to desensitize feelings of embarrassment, shame, or fears they may have about stuttering. This activity also allows children to talk about stuttering with us, parents, and others in different ways.

INSTRUCTIONS FOR USE:

Different kinds of stuttering such as "more tense/less tense," "longer/shorter," "smaller/bigger," etc. are brainstormed in the speech notebook. Next, we attempt to change stuttering, to play around with our speech, with the child in these different ways. The child may teach others how he or she stutters. A "report card" is developed and the child grades the other person (e.g., clinician, parent, teacher, peer) on how well they can stutter (Murphy, 1996). This almost always introduces humor, an important part of the desensitization process. It is important for us to be willing to stutter, to put stuttering in our own mouths, as the child is experiencing it in his.

SHORT-TERM OBJECTIVE:

The child will identify, demonstrate, and teach ___ possible ways of stuttering to clinician or others.

Bobbie
age 9

Ways we can stutter 9/1

short stutters
long stutters
tiny stutters
medium and big stutters
tight stutter
loose stutter

super super super stock
stutters
easy stutters
bouncy stutters

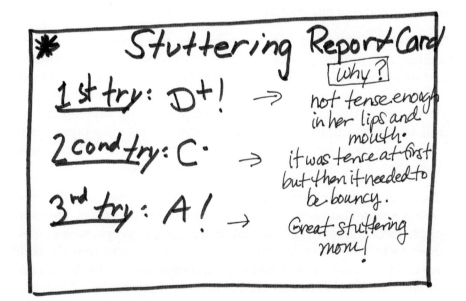

❋ Stuttering Report Card

1st try: D+! → Why? not tense enough in her lips and mouth.

2cond try: C· → it was tense at first but then it needed to be bouncy.

3rd try: A! → Great stuttering mom!

CLINICIAN'S COMMENTS

After brainstorming and practicing different ways to stutter, **Bobbie** developed a report card and graded his mom on her ability to stutter.

Strategy 9: Teaching Others

DESCRIPTION/PURPOSE:

Teaching Others involves a meeting and/or classroom presentation about stuttering, which includes the clinician, child, teacher, parents, and/or other students. The purpose of this strategy is to increase the child's ownership of the problem and develop self-advocacy skills. Children are often more willing to attempt changes in their speech once the teacher or parent "knows" what they are doing. Presenting to the class often reduces the child's need to "hide" the stuttering and may increase overall communication in the classroom (Murphy, 1999).

INSTRUCTIONS FOR USE:

This strategy can be used in many ways. It is critical to suggest it at the right time for a given child. The following suggestions have been useful for many of our clients.

The Meeting: The child, with our help, documents what he wants his teacher (and parents) to know about stuttering *in general* and his stuttering *specifically*. Then, an agenda for the meeting is developed and a plan is negotiated (e.g., who will present certain pieces of information). After the meeting is role-played, we accompany the child to the meeting. Some children have made videotapes about their speech tools and even web pages to educate others. Developing a plan that is interesting to the child is important.

The Peer Presentation: Similar to the Meeting, we help the child develop a presentation about stuttering for the child's class. This may include facts and myths about stuttering, famous people who stutter, speech tools, how we make talking, etc. It is important that the child have a primary role in deciding what information will be shared and how they would wish to execute the presentation.

SHORT-TERM OBJECTIVE:

With the clinician's assistance, the child will develop and execute a plan for a meeting and/or peer presentation about stuttering.

Name: _____

Date: _____

Age: _____

What I Want My _____ to Know About...

What I Want My Stuttering

Stuttering

My Stuttering

What Would Help Me

Pete
Age: 7

When my talking gets hard,
I want my listeners to....

Do	Not Do
eye contact	Make fun of me *make fun of me*
listen	look away *look away*
Stay focused	listen when people interrupt *listen when people interrupt*
and bo not say wait a second	finish words
Wait your turn	Do not remind to use tools *Do not remind to use tools*

CLINICIAN'S COMMENTS

We developed a plan with **Peter** and held a meeting at his school with his teacher and his parents.

August 27

Dear Mrs.

My name is Matt; I am a student in your first hour psychology class. I am writing you this letter to tell you about some personal issues, which may affect my participation in your class. I am part of that 4% of the population that have a stuttering problem. I have had this problem ever since I was little and learned how to put sounds into words to make that taken-for-granted miracle called speech.

I can still talk, mind you, but I just have a more difficult time with it than others. You may have noticed this during our class discussions when I try to explain something and I have a lot more vocal pauses, and interjections like umms and likes, than most other people. This is not because I don't understand the question but rather that I am trying to get through what stutterers call a block. This is one of the main reasons why I rarely volunteer to answer a question or state an opinion during a class discussion; I fear what others may think of me if I stutter. I already have many painful memories of growing up with other students laughing at me during class or snickering during a speech, so as you can probably guess I try to avoid those situations as much as possible. This is not to say that I will just sit like a stump for the whole year and never talk, I will offer my opinion but only if I am feeling especially brave. If I do have a question about something, chances are I'll ask it after class so I avoid embarrassment or discuss something in more detail. Also, if you see that I am having trouble saying a word and if time permits, I ask that you please not finish the sentence of me. (That's a stuttering pet peeve!). I also do not mind doing oral reports in front of the class; in fact I actually like doing them strangely enough so you don't have to worry about that.

I am taking therapy for my stuttering now and am getting better at controlling it but it will never go away completely. I am just a normal kid; I don't have some abnormal brain dysfunction. I ask for your consideration and understanding throughout the year.

Sincerely,

Matt

CLINICIAN'S COMMENTS

Instead of holding a meeting, **Matt** (age 16) decided to write a letter about his speech to his teacher.

Chapter 5

case profiles

In the previous chapters, we have provided methods for assessing children's attitudes and feelings related to their stuttering. We then described strategies we often use to help children achieve these attitudinal changes.

In this chapter, we will use several case studies to illustrate treatment goals and strategies we used based on information from the assessment and the ongoing therapy process. We will focus our examples on four children: John, age 6 who is participating in therapy for the first time; Hailey, age 8, also participating in therapy for her stuttering for the first time; James, age 13, whose parents brought him to therapy hoping this time would have different results; and, Frank, age 15, returning to therapy following a relapse.

Selected examples for each child from the assessment and treatment process will be used to illustrate each child's case history. Remember that the strategies used with each child varied in sequence based on the individual needs of the child.

JOHN

BACKGROUND INFORMATION:

John, age 6, was referred for an evaluation by his parents. He had been stuttering for approximately 18 months but had not yet received services. There was no family history of stuttering, nor any significant events in birth or developmental histories. His other communication skills were within normal limits. John's parents initiated the evaluation process because they had "been waiting for the stuttering to go away, but it hadn't."

ASSESSMENT OF ATTITUDES AND FEELINGS:

During general questioning regarding communication, John commented that he liked to talk but sometimes his speech got "bumpy." With further probing, we asked him how he felt when his speech was bumpy, and he replied that it made him feel nervous because he didn't know why it happened. John also indicated that he was aware of his parents' concern by his statement, "Bumpy speech doesn't bother me, but my mom and dad are worried."

Paper-pencil tasks included **Hands Down** and **Draw Me a Picture** indicated that while he was aware of his stuttering, he didn't seem to view it as a significant negative part of himself.

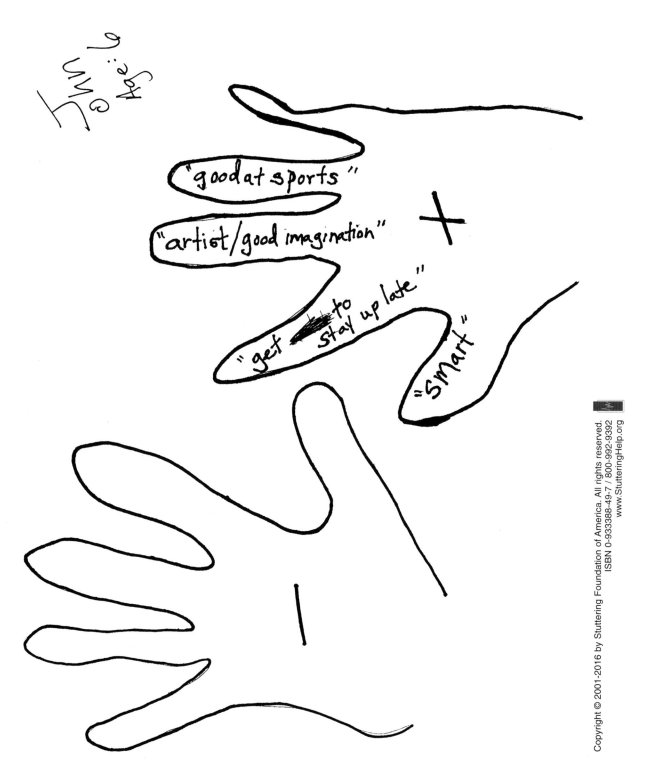

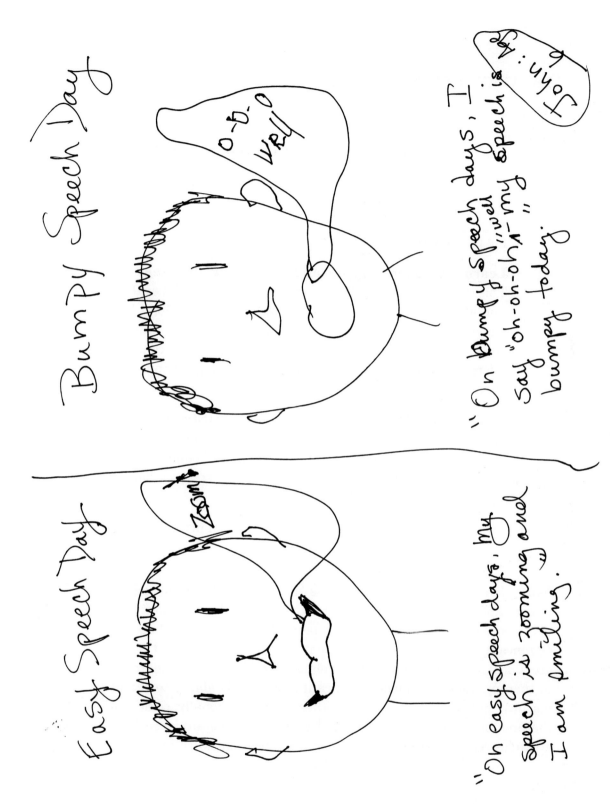

Bumpy Speech Day

"On bumpy speech days, I say "oh-oh-oh-"well" my speech is bumpy today."

John: Age 9

Easy Speech Day

"On easy speech days, my speech is zooming and I am smiling."

TREATMENT PLAN:

Based on assessment data and observations, one of the long term goals for John was to maintain positive attitudes and feelings about communication. This goal was addressed using the following strategies:

- **Creating a Speech Notebook (Strategy 1).** This strategy was used first so that documentation of therapy strategies would be ongoing. John also used his speech notebook to teach his parents and siblings what he was learning in therapy.

- **Learning About Talking and Stuttering (Strategy 2).** This strategy was targeted because, during the initial evaluation and again during the early stages of therapy, John had made several references to feeling unsure about why "bumpy speech was happening." We felt that teaching John concrete information about how speech was made was a good approach to address this issue.

- **Meaningful Topics for Discussion (Strategy 4).** Meaningful topics were identified and expanded upon as issues arose during therapy. One of the most frequent issues for John was that of "mistakes." Using this strategy helped John develop the belief that mistakes are ok.

The following examples are taken from John's speech notebook.

Note: John made excellent progress in therapy. He developed an understanding of the process of speech and learned more about how to better manage his own speech. He became a master at teaching the significant others in his environment about stuttering, and felt a great deal of pride in his ability to relate information he was learning in therapy. John also made significant gains in his ability to accept his own mistakes and those of others. He occasionally comes to therapy for "brush-up" sessions and continues to maintain positive attitudes regarding himself and his communication skills.

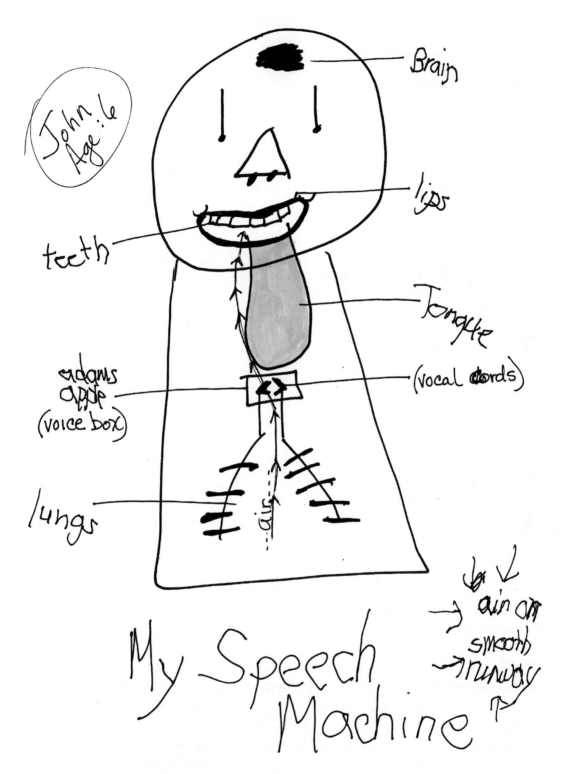

My Speech Machine

Labels in drawing:
- John, Age 6
- Brain
- lips
- teeth
- Tongue
- (vocal cords)
- adams apple (voice box)
- lungs
- air
- air on smooth runway

CLINICIAN'S COMMENTS

John's speech machine was drawn after he'd made a pizza with us. He identified all the parts he uses to make talking.

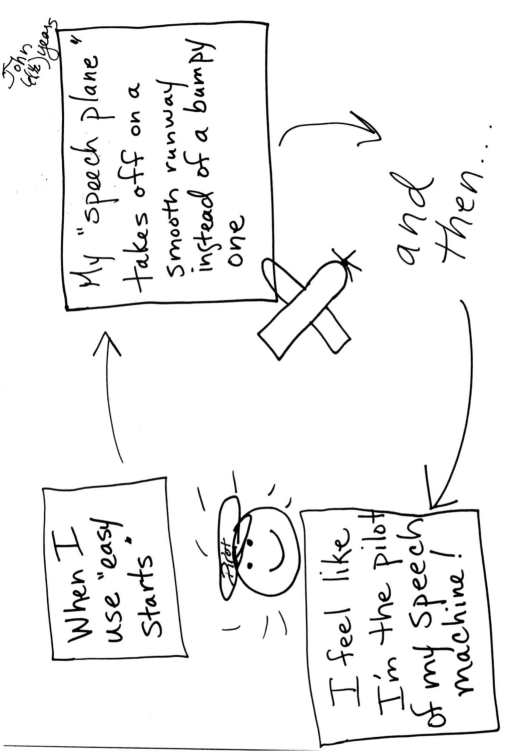

138

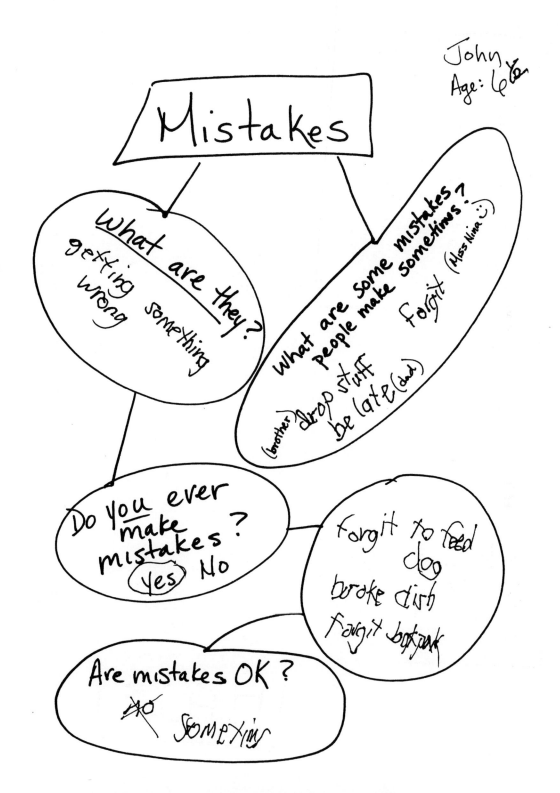

John
Age: 6½

Mistakes

What are they?
getting something wrong

What are some mistakes?
people make sometimes?
(brother) drop stuff
be late (dad)
forgit (Miss Nina :))

Do you ever make mistakes?
(Yes) No

forgit to feed dog
broke dish
forgit bakpak

Are mistakes OK?
NO somethin

HAILEY

BACKGROUND INFORMATION:

Hailey entered therapy for stuttering in third grade. Her developmental and medical histories were insignificant. There was no history of stuttering in the family. Hailey had been stuttering for one year, and had received treatment for articulation in second grade. Hailey's mother reported that she was exhibiting some word avoidances and frustration. She had also observed significant blocks accompanied by facial tension and the use of her upper body to get her words out. She had observed Hailey giving up during attempts to say words on numerous occasions, with Hailey announcing, "I can't say it."

ASSESSMENT OF ATTITUDES AND FEELINGS:

When Hailey was questioned about her speech in a general way, she stated that she liked talking mostly to her friends about horses, but that it wasn't always easy for her to communicate. When she was asked if she wanted to change something, she said, "Just to make it come out smoother," and called the problem "easy bouncing." She did not report any specific situational speaking fears. Further probing revealed the following:

- a description of easy bouncing as when her words were bumpy and wouldn't come out

- it happened more at home than at school, and sometimes with her friends;

- when it did happen, she tried to push it out as best she could; and,

- she felt frustrated because some children had started to mimic her talking at school

The paper-pencil task **What's True for You** was given to Hailey during the initial evaluation. Her responses on this task and her answers during questioning/probing suggested that negative attitudes and feelings were beginning to develop. These perceptions were further supported by observations of Hailey. She exhibited nonverbal behaviors such as loss of eye contact or shifts in body position, as well as word avoidance or substitutions. Although these behaviors occurred infrequently, it was our feeling that they signaled the need to address her attitudes and feelings as soon as possible.

Parent report indicated that they were at a "loss" for how to help Hailey with her talking. They felt that she was aware of the problem and that her frustration was increasing. They were also concerned about how the stuttering would affect her self esteem.

Hailey's teacher felt that she was continuing to communicate regularly in the classroom, although she had noticed more blocking and loss of eye contact. She did not feel that Hailey demonstrated outward concern about her speech.

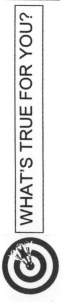

WHAT'S TRUE FOR YOU?

Name: _Taylor_
Date: _2/__
Age: _2nd grade_

Read each statement. Circle the number that best describes what's true for you.

1. I wish I could talk like other kids.

1   ④   7
No Way   Sometimes   I totally agree

2. Some people are hard to talk to.

①   4   7
No Way   Sometimes   I totally agree

3. I talk openly about my speech with my parents.

1   4   ⑦
No Way   Sometimes   I totally agree

4. I am a good talker.

1   4   ⑦
No Way   Sometimes   I totally agree

5. I like to talk.

1   4   ⑦
No Way   Sometimes   I totally agree

6. Sometimes I do things so I won't have trouble talking (like not talking or changing words or thoughts).

1   ④   7
No Way   Sometimes   I totally agree

like when
I get stuck in second grade.
"I didn't want to get stuck."

7. I have sounds that are hard for me to say.

1   4   ⑦ _The "l" and "s" sounds_
No Way   Sometimes   I totally agree

8. It's O.K. to have trouble talking sometimes.

①   4   7
No Way   Sometimes   I totally agree

9. I have gotten teased about my speech.

1   4   ⑦
No Way   Sometimes   I totally agree

10. I don't like having trouble talking.

1   4   ⑦
No Way   Sometimes   I totally agree

11. I want to improve the way I talk.

1   4   ⑦
No Way   Sometimes   I totally agree

Chmela & Reardon, 1999

13

TREATMENT PLAN:

Based on the assessment data and observations, one of the long-term goals for Hailey was to develop positive attitudes and feelings related to stuttering. This goal was addressed using the following strategies:

- **Creating a Speech Notebook (Strategy 1).** Creating a notebook was implemented so that concepts learned could be reviewed and Hailey could teach others about what she was learning in therapy.

- **Learning About Talking and Stuttering (Strategy 2).** This strategy was chosen so that we could provide Hailey with an understanding of what was happening when she had trouble talking. Creating the foundation of "making choices" about changing her speech was also important.

- **Experimenting with Stuttering (Strategy 8).** This strategy was implemented because of Hailey's developing response to tense moments of stuttering.

- **Teaching Others (Strategy 9).** This strategy was incorporated by having Hailey meet with her teacher. Hailey also chose to do a classroom presentation about stuttering at a later time in therapy.

- **Meaningful Topics for Discussion (Strategy 4).** Meaningful topics were highlighted and explored in the speech notebook as appropriate.

- **Problem-Solving Plans (Strategy 5).** Problem-solving plans were developed as needed in the speech notebook, especially to help Hailey create solutions for teasing she was experiencing at school.

Note: Hailey has made excellent progress in therapy. The careful consideration of negative attitudes that appeared to be in the developing stages was important. The above therapy plan along with the relationship created with Hailey resulted in a quick turn around of such attitudes. Hailey learned to increase her fluency and change her stuttering by using a variety of tools. She increased her understanding of speech tools by diagramming them in her speech notebook either using webs or concept maps. Such exercises helped Hailey understand what the tools were, how to use them, and why they helped. This increased understanding ultimately improved her attitudes about stuttering. Validating her frustration and encouraging her for becoming responsible for her "speech machine" were important components of Hailey's treatment. Presently, we are working on maintaining Hailey's positive attitudes and improving her ability to transfer skills learned in therapy to other environments.

The following examples are excerpts taken from Hailey's speech notebook.

Must Have: to make Pizza Hailey 2/20

3rd grade

1. Pizza dough : crust
2. sauce
3. cheese

Choices:
pepperoin
sausage
mushroom
peppers
Onions
bacon
pineapple
anchovies

A. You must have certain ingredients.
B. You must make it in a certain order or way.
C. There are lots of choices.

CLINICIAN'S COMMENTS

During learning about talking, we made a real pizza. The pizza helped **Hailey** understand how we make talking and the importance of making choices for changing how we talk.

Hailey's Points about Pizza:

2/20

1) The more you do something the easier it is, i.e., the more you make pizza the more you know how to do it.

2) You need to be prepared. You need the hotmits.

3) You need to pay attention.(or you'll get burned)

4) It's easier to put the cheese on with the your hand 'cause you have more control.

5) It's hard to remember to use the hotmits (when you go to cut the pizza)

6) If Miss Kristin helps me cut the pizza I can learn how to do it by myself.

7) It's easier to make this pizza if I take my time.

8) It's o.k. if you make a mistake.

CLINICIAN'S COMMENTS

Hailey made these comments during the pizza activity. We listed them in her speech notebook and discussed them later in therapy. As you can see, they related to all aspects of stuttering therapy!

Must Have: to make talking

jaw

tongue

throat

brain

lips

teeth

voice box

vocal cords

lungs

diaphragm

My speech Workspop
2/27

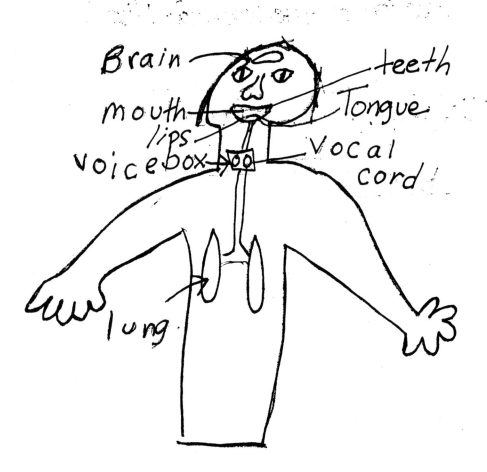

Brain
mouth
lips
Voicebox
teeth
Tongue
Vocal
cord
lung

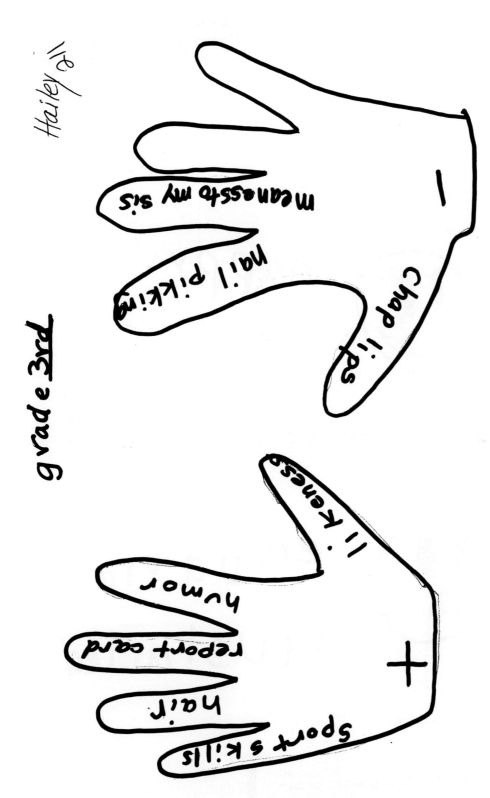

Hailey 8"

grade 3rd

Humor
report card
hair
Sport skills
likeness
+

Meaness to my sis
Nail Picking
Chap lips
−

CLINICIAN'S COMMENTS

These paper-pencil tasks were administered as treatment progressed. **Hailey** was able to express her negative feelings about talking, although we perceived positive attitudes overall about herself and communication in general.

Name: *Hailey*
Date: 2/1/00

What does your face look like.........

On an easy talking day?????????????

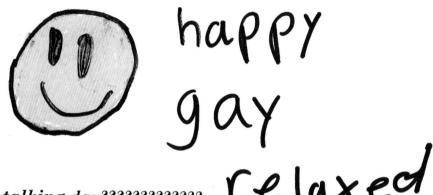

happy
gay
relaxed

On a hard talking day?????????????

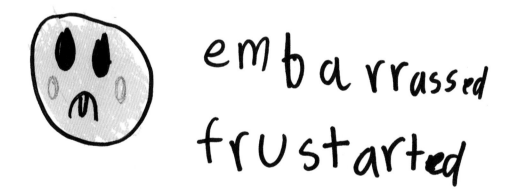

embarrassed
frustarted

Appropriate for ages five years and older

Name: *Hailey*
Date: 2/1/00

Draw me a picture of.................................

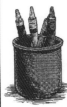

Who: your family
What: talking
Where: at the dinner table

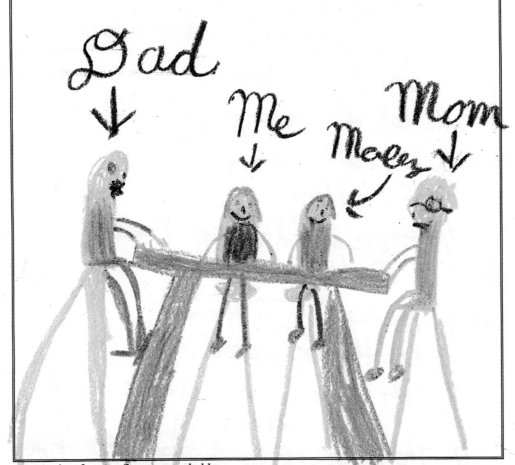

Appropriate for ages five years and older

CLINICIAN'S COMMENTS

Hailey's parents and her sister were involved in her treatment on a regular basis. We worked on reflective listening and turn taking. Her parents learned to make observations about Hailey's speech, which allowed them to talk about it in a nonjudgmental way.

What I Know about Stuttering: (so far!)

3/2

1. It's o.k. to stutter.
2. Stuttering is no one's fault.
3. Sometimes when you stutter your speech machine doesn't do what it's suppose to.
4. Lots of famous people stutter.
5. We don't know the cause of stuttering
6. There are different kinds of stuttering.
7. No two people stutter exactly the same.
8. Lots of people are curious about stuttering.
9. There's lots of things people who stutter can do to talk easier.

CLINICIAN'S COMMENTS

Things **Hailey** learned about stuttering were listed in the notebook and reviewed consistently. We also researched myths about stuttering, and famous people who stutter.

Question of the week for Miss Kristin:

Did you stutter when you were my age?

Question from Hailey to Miss Kristin:

Are you born with stuttering or can you get it later on in your life?

5/1

? for: What don't you
like about speech tools?

Sometimes they don't
work how I what ~~them~~
them too.
           Like.... when I
get stuck and I can't
stop.

"I'm learning
tools"

eye contact
easy beginning
cancelling
chunking
wait time

therefore →

I should not
ever get bumpy
again

OR

I am getting
better at managing my
bumpy speech when it
happens

CLINICIAN'S COMMENTS

We explored **Hailey's** reluctance to use speech tools by asking her a Question of the Week, combined with Meaningful Topic for Discussion. This activity gave Hailey the opportunity to communicate her frustration with stuttering.

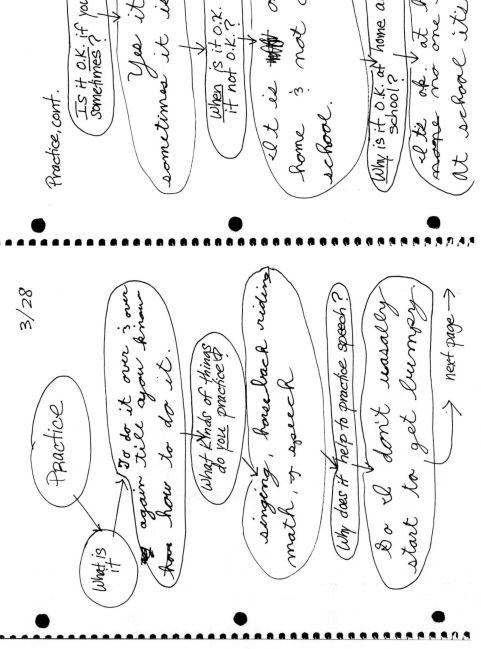

Practice, cont.   P.2

Is it o.k. if you get bumpy sometimes?

Yes it is; sometimes it is not.

When is it o.k. and when is it not o.k.?

It is o.k. at home & not o.k. at school.

Why is it o.k. at home and not o.k. at school?

It is o.k. at home because no one repeats me. (repeats) At school it's not o.k.?

3/28

Practice

What is it

To do it over & over again till you know how to do it.

What kinds of things do you practice?

singing, horseback riding, math, & speech

Why does it help to practice speech?

So I don't usually start to get bumpy.

→ next page →

CLINICIAN'S COMMENTS

As therapy progressed, **Hailey** was having difficulty following through with home practice. "Practice" was identified as a Meaningful Topic for Discussion. Hailey's responses during this activity led to a discussion about a classroom presentation.

→ Maybe... (A) they are confused? (B) they are mean? (C) they want your attention?

I pick A.

What could we do about it?

Maybe you could come to my class 3. talk to my class

Will you help me?

Yes I will help yours!

YOU ARE A VERY SMART THINKER!

Practice →cont: P.3

→ Because some kids kids copy me.

Where in school are kids copying you? What do you mean "copy you?"

Kids copy me in the class room. What I mean by copy is if I do bumpy speech they to repeat me in bumpy speech

Why do you think they copy you?

Maybe they think it's funny fuennoy.

Name: **Hailey**
Date: 4/1/00
Age: **8**

What I Want My I E A C H E R to Know About...

Stuttering	My Stuttering	What Would Help Me
1.) It's O.K. to stutter.	1.) I only stutter sometimes.	1.) Don't interrupt me.
2.) stuttering is no ones fault.	2.) I'm embarrassed sometimes.	2.) Keep calling on me.
3.) It's sometimes how I talk.	3.) talking is pretty easy at school.	3.) If I get stuck look at me, let me finish; don't say my words.
4.) I was made that way?	4.) Sometimes I put an "a" in front of a word ⟶	4.) Help me with tools
5.) More boys stutter than Girls.	5.) if I am stuck. ⟶	5.) I like talking in school.

Appropriate for ages 8 years and older

Copyright © 2001-2016 by Stuttering Foundation of America. All rights reserved.
ISBN 0-933388-49-7 / 800-992-9392
www.StutteringHelp.org

JAMES

BACKGROUND INFORMATION:

James, age 13, had been enrolled in speech therapy since first grade. Prior therapy had been inconsistent, and both James and his parents were frustrated by his lack of progress. The focus of past therapy had primarily been on speech behaviors, with little attention given to attitudes and feelings. There was a family history of stuttering on the father's side, and James was diagnosed in fifth grade as having Attention Deficit Disorder and was on medication.

ASSESSMENT OF ATTITUDES AND FEELINGS:

When asked why he was coming to speech at this time, James responded "I am really frustrated with my speech right now." During further probing, James talked openly about significant sound, word, and situational avoidances. In addition, we observed a lack of eye contact and that he used his hand to partially cover his mouth during moments of stuttering. From his conversation and body language, we got the impression that he had low self-confidence and high anxiety about communication.

What's True for You, Here's What I Think, and **Count Me Out** were the paper-pencil evaluation tasks we chose to use with James. His responses indicated that he didn't know much about typical speech production or stuttering, that he had strong fears and avoidances associated with stuttering. We perceived that he was highly motivated to make changes. These responses confirmed what James had shared during questioning and probing.

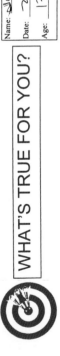

WHAT'S TRUE FOR YOU?

Name: James
Date: 2-2
Age: 13

Read each statement. Circle the number that best describes what's true for you.

1. I wish I could talk like other kids.

1   4   7
No Way   Sometimes   I totally agree

2. Some people are hard to talk to.

"Authority figures on bad speech days"

1   4   7
No Way   Sometimes   I totally agree

3. I talk openly about my speech with my parents.

1   4   7
No Way   Sometimes   I totally agree

4. I am a good talker.

1   4   7
No Way   Sometimes   I totally agree

5. I like to talk.

1   4   7
No Way   Sometimes   I totally agree

6. Sometimes I do things so I won't have trouble talking (like not talking or changing words or thoughts).

1   4   7
No Way   Sometimes   I totally agree

7. I have sounds that are hard for me to say.

"s, m, w and b words"

1   4   7
No Way   Sometimes   I totally agree

8. It's O.K. to have trouble talking sometimes.

1   4   7
No Way   Sometimes   I totally agree

9. I have gotten teased about my speech.

1   4   7
No Way   Sometimes   I totally agree

10. I don't like having trouble talking.

1   4   7
No Way   Sometimes   I totally agree

11. I want to improve the way I talk.

"I'm frustrated now and really want to improve"

1   4   7
No Way   Sometimes   I totally agree

Appropriate for ages 8 years and older

Name: James
Date: 2-2
Age: 13

Here's What I Think *Interview*

1. I am here because "I stutter"

2. In previous therapy I learned "to talk slower, stretch my speech, use eye contact when stuttering."

3. Some thing(s) I liked about my previous speech therapy were they (5 different speech teachers) helped me learn what to do."

4. Some things(s) I did not like about my previous speech therapy were "cut down on school time - had extra homework"

5. My parents were involved in my previous therapy.   (circle one) "Sort-of"
   Yes   No   If Yes, How? Parent conference days

6. I want to come to speech now.   (circle one) (Yes)   No
   Why? "It can help"

7. A question I have about stuttering is "how can I be more steady at controlling it?"

8. I feel comfortable/uncomfortable (circle one) "Sometimes" talking to my parents about my speech because "we don't usually talk about it."

Appropriate for Ages 9 and Older

Name: James
Date:
Age: 13

"COUNT ME OUT"

Many people may avoid speaking in situations because they think they may stutter.

Read each statement below.
Check whether you would *Always, Sometimes* or *Never* avoid the situation.

	Always	*Sometimes*	*Never*
☐ Ordering for myself in a restaurant	X		
☐ Talking with friends			X
☐ Asking for a date		X	
☐ Calling a store for information	X		
☐ Talking to an authority figure		X	
☐ Giving directions		X	
☐ Talking to my parents			X
☐ Talking to a store clerk	X		
☐ Answering/talking on the phone		X	
☐ Giving a speech in class	X		
☐ Reading aloud		X	

Appropriate for ages 12 years and older

TREATMENT PLAN:

The long-term goal for James was to develop more positive attitudes and feelings about stuttering, communication, and self. Treatment activities were presented in the following sequence:

- **Creating a Speech Notebook (Strategy 1).** James created a speech notebook to track concepts and progress in therapy. The notebook was reviewed consistently throughout therapy so James could understand the relationships between attitudes and speech behaviors.

- **Learning About Talking and Stuttering (Strategy 2).** This strategy was essential for James. Years of therapy with multiple therapists had left him confused regarding the facts of stuttering and speech production. He both wanted and needed straightforward information.

- **Meaningful Topics for Discussion (Strategy 4).** This strategy was used periodically throughout therapy to explore issues as they arose.

- **Experimenting with Stuttering (Strategy 8).** Experimenting with stuttering helped desensitize James to the "out of control" feelings he was experiencing during tense stuttering moments. Experimenting also provided opportunities for James to discuss stuttering with his parents in a more open and comfortable manner.

- **Changing My Thinking (Strategy 6).** This strategy was implemented as we discovered that James consistently "beat himself up" during stuttering moments. By identifying and learning to change his thinking, James began to view himself and his stuttering in more positive ways.

- **Developing Speech Hierarchies (Strategy 7).** Developing a hierarchy was an important component of therapy because it allowed James to address the fear he was experiencing in many speaking situations. We discovered that the degree of fear James felt was in direct proportion to the degree of avoidance he exhibited. James first learned about fear and how it related to his stuttering, then developed a series of steps using a Worry Ladder to manage the fear by gradually progressing through the hierarchy he created.

- **Problem-Solving Plans (Strategy 5).** Plans were created as necessary throughout therapy.

Note: James made excellent progress in therapy but experienced two short relapses during his maintenance period. James' problem-solving skills helped him work through both of these difficult times. James now comes for therapy "tune ups" when he feels he needs them and attends group therapy sessions one time per month.

The following examples were taken from James' speech notebook.

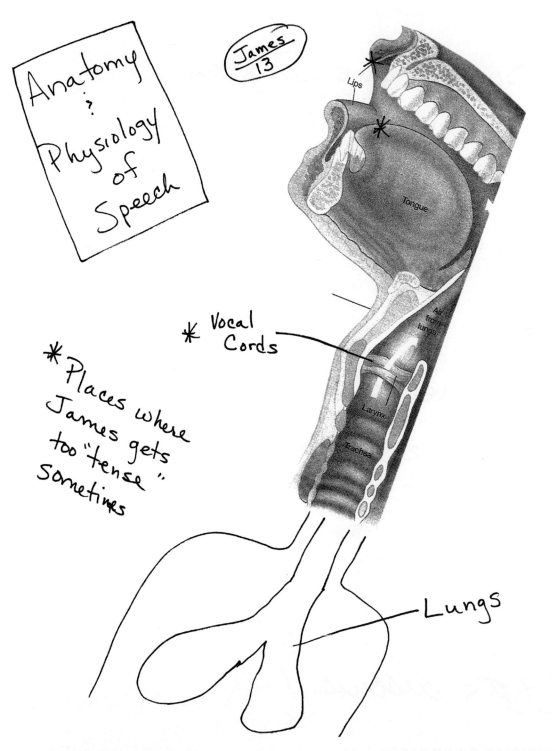

Anatomy & Physiology of Speech

James 13

Lips

Tongue

Air from lungs

* Vocal Cords

Larynx

Trachea

* Places where James gets too "tense" Sometimes

Lungs

Some things I know   James
about Stuttering are: 13

1.) There are good + bad days.
2.) There are things I can do to help my speech.

Some questions I
have about stuttering
are:

1.) Why do ~~xxxx~~ some people stutter + others don't?
2.) Do people ever stop stuttering?

Let's discuss!!

CLINICIAN'S COMMENTS

James brought in two Questions of the Week that were then used as a springboard for Meaningful Topics for Discussion.

<u>Let's experiment</u> :

James
14

- <u>L</u>ist the ways we can
  stutter . . . . prolongation

  repetitions ⟨ Sounds
             syllables
             words

  blocks ⟨ Hard
        regular
        extra long

- <u>L</u>et's try some together
  & see how we do . . . .
  ↓   ↓

<u>D</u>ad's grades | <u>N</u>ina's grades

- √ – – √ + + | + √ – – + + +

(√ = almost
  + = good
  – = no way)

CLINICIAN'S COMMENTS

James experimented with different ways to stutter. He taught his dad how to stutter and "graded" him using a report card.

Copyright © 2001-2016 by Stuttering Foundation of America. All rights reserved.
ISBN 0-933388-49-7 / 800-992-9392
www.StutteringHelp.org

Name: James
Date:
Age: 13

Changing My Thinking

What we think can affect how we feel and what we do! List below some thoughts you say in your head that make you feel bad about yourself. Change those hurtful thoughts into helpful thoughts, or things you say in your head that may make you feel better.

Helpful Thinking

① I will answer this question by taking my time

② Some times I stutter when I read out loud.

③ I will have friends in high school like I do in grade school

Hurtful Thinking

① I am going to stutter if I answer this question.

② I always stutter when I read in class.

③ No body in high school will like me if I stutter.

Intervention Strategy
Appropriate for ages 10 years and older

CLINICIAN'S COMMENTS

James identified negative thoughts he had about stuttering. Each thought was addressed and changed into a helpful or more positive thought.

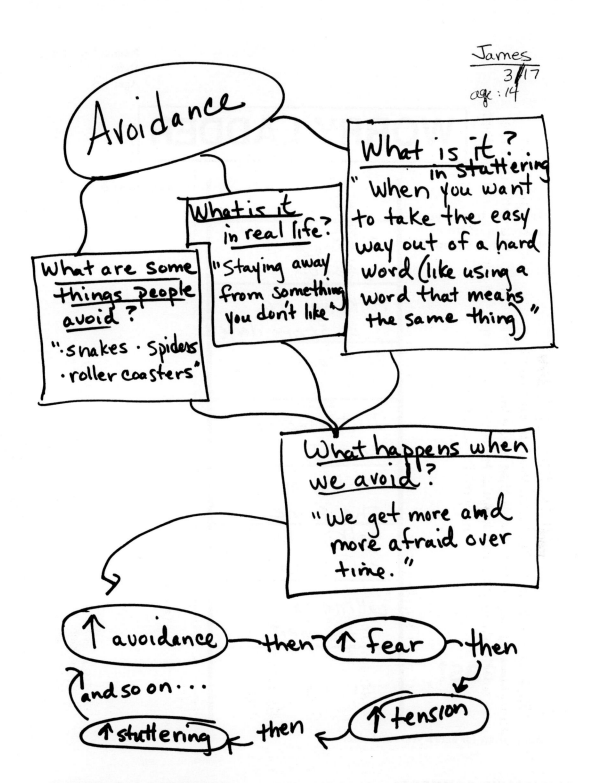

James
3/17
age: 14

Avoidance

What is it?
in stuttering
"When you want
to take the easy
way out of a hard
word (like using a
word that means
the same thing)"

What is it
in real life?
"Staying away
from something
you don't like"

What are some
things people
avoid?
"·snakes · spiders
·roller coasters"

What happens when
we avoid?
"We get more and
more afraid over
time."

↑ avoidance — then — ↑ fear — then
and so on...
↑ stuttering — then — ↑ tension

Name: James
Date:
Age: 13

WORRY LADDER

most

Write the things you worry about from the least to the most.

giving a speech
talking to a store clerk
giving directions
Introducing friends
talking on the phone
talking to kids I don't know
calling a stranger

least

Appropriate for ages 8 years and older

CLINICIAN'S COMMENTS

A Worry Ladder was used to help **James** create a hierarchy of feared speaking situations.

FRANK

BACKGROUND INFORMATION:

Frank began stuttering at age four. There was no significant medical or developmental history or family history of stuttering. Frank had received therapy during his kindergarten year, and then from third to fourth grade. Treatment at that time was successful, and involved teaching him general fluency shaping procedures as well as strategies to maintain positive attitudes and feelings about stuttering, communication, and self. At the time of the current referral, Frank was 15 and his mother was concerned about how he'd been "freezing up" during communication. She noted increased tension including eye blinking and facial movements. She was concerned about his not being motivated to work on his speech and resume practicing.

ASSESSMENT OF ATTITUDES AND FEELINGS:

When asked why he returned to therapy, Frank stated, "because my speech is falling apart." Further probing revealed that his stuttering had been fairly mild for the past several years but in recent months talking had become more difficult. He stated that several peers had mentioned his problem at school, and that may have triggered his relapse. He further shared that he didn't remember his speech tools and that he was not as comfortable participating in class. He said that at times when he stuttered, he felt embarrassed and frustrated. He also said that although he wouldn't avoid giving a speech, he was very worried about it.

Paper-pencil tasks included **Here's What I Think** and **What Pops.** It was evident from these tasks that although Frank was not necessarily avoiding, he had developed some negative attitudes and feelings about his stuttering problem and communication. Talking in some situations was particularly difficult.

Parent report further indicated that Frank didn't appear to be significantly "bothered" by his stuttering. His mother stated that she

171

often told him to stop and start over and that he seemed to be frustrated by this advice.

Frank's teachers reported that he occasionally participated in class. His history teacher noted that Frank often hesitated before giving an answer. He also mentioned that there would be several presentation assignments coming up in his class. Additionally, he noted that Frank didn't seem upset about his speech in school.

TREATMENT PLAN:

One long-term goal for Frank was to develop more positive attitudes and feelings about stuttering and communication. Because of Frank's love of the computer, it was often used to implement the various strategies during treatment. The following strategies were used with Frank.

- **Creating a Speech Notebook (Strategy 1).** Frank's speech notebook was created on a computer disk rather than in notebook form. A hard copy of each entry was printed at each session and kept in his treatment folder.

- **Learning About Talking and Stuttering (Strategy 2).** This was critical for Frank. Time was spent helping Frank understand the mechanics of speech production and the concept of choosing to modify speech in different ways.

- **Question/Statement of the Week (Strategy 3).** This strategy was implemented in order to discuss issues related to stuttering. It also served as a vehicle by which Frank and his parents could discuss stuttering.

- **Meaningful Topics for Discussion (Strategy 4).** Meaningful topics were explored when appropriate.

- **Teaching Others (Strategy 9).** This involved Frank directing a meeting with a teacher of his choice. Frank also successfully taught his parents about his speech tools and other information throughout the treatment process.

- **Experimenting with Stuttering (Strategy 8).** This strategy allowed Frank to desensitize to the body response he was experiencing during a stuttering moment (e.g., increasing tension, breaking eye contact, rolling his eyes). Frank developed the ability to maintain eye contact during stuttering. This facilitated an overall decrease in tension and stuttering in an easier way. These changes ultimately had a positive effect on Frank's attitudes about stuttering and communication.

- **Problem-Solving Plans (Strategy 5).** Problem-solving plans were created when necessary.

Note: Frank made good progress in therapy. He is continuing to work on his speech independently, although he attends therapy every other month for maintenance purposes. The following examples are taken from his speech disk.

Name: Frank
Date: 4/1
Age: 15

Here's What I Think

1. I am here because _of my speech_

2. In previous therapy I learned _speech tools_

3. Some things I liked about my previous speech therapy were _It helped me for_ _a while. My teacher was nice._

4. Some things I did not like about my previous speech therapy were _It didn't last —_ _it wore off._

5. My parents were involved in my previous therapy.   (circle one)

   Yes   (No)   If yes, How? _____

6. I want to come to speech now   (circle one)   (yes)   no
   Why? _My speech is falling apart and I'm starting to_ _get nervous about talking in some situations._

7. A question I have about stuttering is _why does it change over time?_

8. I feel comfortable (uncomfortable) (circle one) talking to my parents about my speech because _I think they think I'm not trying or don't care._

Appropriate for ages 9 years and older

WHAT "POPS?"

Name: Frank   Date: 4/1

Complete the sentences below with the first thing that comes to your mind. There are no right or wrong answers.

1. Most of all I want... *to do well in school*
2. I'm afraid... *rollercoasters*
3. A sister or brother should... *help you*
4. My father always.... *travels*
5. People are always... *friendly*
6. I know I can... *do anything*
7. I hate... *when I'm time pressured*
8. I worry about... *my speech*
9. My family... *gets along*
10. I wish I could stop... *blocking so much*
11. There is nothing... *I like about homework*
12. I wish... *I could travel more*
13. Mother and I... *fight sometimes*
14. When I get mad... *I go in my room*
15. When I grow up... *I want a good job*
16. At school... *I work alot*
17. It hurts when... *people tease you*
18. People shouldn't... *tease*
19. I want to know... *more about stuttering*
20. I will never... *fail at math*
21. My friends think I... *nice*
22. I get mad when... *I'm late*
23. My mother never... *stays mad*
24. At home... *I stutter alot*
25. Other kids... *a nice*
26. I just can't... *stop stuttering on my own*
27. I'm different because... *stutter*
28. My best friend... *is cool*
29. My favorite... *subject is science*
30. This year... *is almost over*

32

Original Paper Developed by Chmela & Reardon, 1995

Speech Journal

April 26

The Speech Process parallels making a pizza

What you must have.........the order or sequence of how it its put together...choices
1. Crust   Vocal Chords
2. Sauce   tongue
3. Cheese   lips
                  mouth
                  lungs
                  brain
                  diaphragm
                  voice box

1. respiration
2. phonation
3. articulation

Pizza Choices: Talking Choices:
pepperoni   fast talking
sausage   regular
olives   slowly
peppers   hard
ham   soft
pineapple   easy onsets
onion   phrasing
mushrooms   resisting time pressure
anchovies   canceling
                                  pull-outs
                                  easy bouncing

Tension: When our body becomes stressed, tight
Stresses on the speech system:
being excited
put on the spot
talking fast
tired
trying not to stutter
worrying
feeling bad about something and keeping it inside

Goal of Speech Therapy now: To not ever stutter again (no) To be the best communicator possible (yes) Includes:

What we do when we talk	What we think about it	How we feel about it

CLINICIAN'S COMMENTS

Frank's therapy began with learning about talking. The concept of "being tense" was highlighted as a Meaningful Topic for Discussion. The goal of therapy was also discussed.

May 11

Question of the Week: (from Mrs. Chmela to Frank)
What does being a good communicator involve?
Listening
being concise
thinking about what you're saying
being clear
gestures
body
eye contact
interesting voice and intonation
expressions
fluency

Interesting point: Fluency is 10% of my ability to be a good communicator

June 10

Question from Frank to Mrs. Chmela:
Why is easier onset easier to use with vowels?
Why do people stutter in different ways?

June 17

Question from mom to Frank: Do you think you handle your speech problem in a positive way?

C L I N I C I A N ' S   C O M M E N T S

Several Questions of the Week were generated in different ways. Increasing **Frank's** understanding of stuttering was an important and ongoing part of his treatment.

Meaningful Topic: "Escape"

What does it mean?

To get away from something, to run , to hide; such as danger

Some things I do to "escape" from stuttering:
1. look down
2. use garbage words before the word like "uhm, uh, like..."
3. clear my throat
4. stalling
5. pretend like I forgot what it was called

These keep me running from instead of facing my stuttering.

Do you ever talk about your stuttering or mention it as a way to cope with a tough speaking moment?
I did not want to because it felt kind of embarrassing to mention it in front of someone.

It felt embarrassing because:
I have never done it before and I don't feel comfortable talking about my stuttering.

And you don't feel comfortable talking about it because:
I am uncomfortable with my stuttering.

Ways to get comfortable with stuttering:

> **learn speech tools**
> **meet others that stutter**
> **realize what stuttering is: something you do with your mouth sometimes**
> **taking risks: doing things that you don't usually do or have never done before.**

CLINICIAN'S COMMENTS

Hiding stuttering (i.e., escaping) was explored as a Meaningful Topic of Discussion. This was an issue that came up in response to **Frank's** mother's observations about his stuttering at home. Modeling for his mother ways to make speech observations (the first step of encouraging praise) was helpful. Frank's mother improved in her ability to learn to talk about his stuttering in increasingly nonjudgmental ways.

Building Hierarchies:
levels of steps of a process that graduate from easier to more difficult:

Goal: to make phone calls myself
Specific situation: call my mom at home and my dad at work

Step 5: **Do it from home/school**

Step 4: **Call Dad from Mrs. C's office**

Step 3: **Steps 1 & 2 with mom**

Step 2: **Use 2 phones in Mrs. C's house**

Step 1: **Use 2 phones in Mrs. C's office**

CLINICIAN'S COMMENTS

A speech hierarchy was developed to help **Frank** desensitize his anxiety about making phone calls.

9/14/99

Things I have noticed about my speech since I got to highschool:
I seem to have more trouble talking with teachers than with friends, like when I ask a teacher a question.

Answers to questions from Brad (from when we played the game together):
1. Were you nervous when we played the game? *No, not at all.*
2. What was the hardest part for you when you were playing the game with someone you didn't know? *Nothing. I just wanted to play it.*
3. Do you have trouble keeping eye contact when you talk in general? *I did, but it's getting better because I have been working on it.*
4. Do you have trouble looking at people when you are stuttering? *I do, but I know how important it is to keep eye contact so I have been working on it. Eye contact helped me with the dean at my high school when I got an unexcused absence by mistake. I think by keeping eye contact it made me look confident and honest.*
5. Are you afraid to use techniques in front of others? *I don't know if I'm afraid. Sometimes I just forget and other times I just feel awkward. I have some advice for you: Keep eye contact. It helps you and your audience a lot when you keep eye contact. Also having good friends helps you a lot with your stuttering. They do not care when you stutter.*

CLINICIAN'S COMMENTS

Frank answered questions from another child who stuttered that he met at a group therapy session.

9/21/99

Meeting Agenda with Social Studies Teacher:

I. Purpose of meeting: to tell you about stuttering and about my goals in your classroom.

II. Basic Facts about stuttering

III. My Stuttering:
age three it began
I've been working on my speech
good days and bad days
I like contributing in class but sometimes I don't because I'm uncomfortable

IV. When I stutter you might see me:
I might get really stuck and nothing will come out
I might use "uhm" or "uh" because I am trying to get through a block.

V. When I stutter it would be helpful if:
You would let me finish; sometimes it might look like I don't know the answer when I really do.

VI. I've chosen your class to work on my speech.

VII. I am learning tools and have developed speech goals for your classroom.

VIII. When we have a presentation, I may want to practice it with you alone in the classroom once before I give it.

CLINICIAN'S COMMENTS

Frank developed an agenda and directed a meeting with his history teacher. He chose to meet with this teacher because he had to make a presentation in the class. After this meeting, Frank shared his surprise at how interested his teacher had been in stuttering. He also stated that it was easier for him to communicate in class after this experience.

2/9/99

Problem Solving Plan: I am having more trouble talking

Possible factors:

Loss of sleep..............tired speech mechanism doesn't work as well
School work stress: finals and project........increased stress leads to increased tension and stuttering
No speech check-ins..............stop thinking about speech, makes it harder to manage
Reactions to stuttering..............your stuttering gets bigger and harder to handle
Not talking about it appropriately..........may cause frustration to build up, more stuttering

1. Problem: I am noticing a little more trouble with my stuttering
2. I feel frustrated because I am stuttering more and I want to manage my speech better.
3. Possible solutions:
   get on better sleep routine
   have more consistent speech check-ins
   monitor reactions to stuttering
   talk about it with mom or dad
   be more proactive instead of reactive: practice
4. If/then..all of these solutions would be to my benefit.
5. Come to speech next week and re-evaluate how it's going.

CLINICIAN'S COMMENTS

A problem-solving plan was created several months later during a time when **Frank** was phasing out of weekly therapy. Learning the process of problem-solving was important for Frank. Hopefully in the future, this skill will enable him to manage his stuttering independently.

IN CONCLUSION...

In reading this book, we hope you have seen how feelings and beliefs about stuttering and communication can be as much a part of the stuttering problem for a school-age child as the disfluency itself.

Remember that stuttering is a complex problem; therefore, the feelings and beliefs that accompany it are not only complex but also different for each child. As you begin to work with children who stutter, consider the three important points mentioned in chapter one.

First, the quantity and quality of stuttering behaviors may not be in direct relationship to the intensity of the negative feelings and beliefs the child is experiencing.

Second, children and families differ in the way they think and feel about stuttering.

Third, children vary in their ability to understand and talk about their feelings and beliefs.

Sharpen your own communication skills by learning to validate and encourage children. This is a critical part of the stuttering therapy process. These assessment and treatment tools can help you document important aspects of the problem as well as outcomes of therapy, resulting in the child's increased participation in the classroom and positive changes in how the child views stuttering.

Our hope is that you will be able to employ these tools to help the children you work with to become the best communicators possible.

References

Andre, S., & Guitar, B. (1979). The A-19 Scale for children who stutter. In Peters, T., & Guitar, B. (1991). *Stuttering: An integrated approach to its nature and treatment.* Baltimore, MD: Williams & Wilkins and in (1999) *Stuttering: An Integration of Contemporary Therapies,* Memphis, TN: Stuttering Foundation of America.

Briggs, D. C. (1975). *Your child's self esteem: The key to life.* New York: Doubleday and Company.

Campbell, J. H. (1998). Therapy for school-age children who stutter. Presented to the Workshop for Stuttering Specialists, Northwestern University, Evanston, IL.

Coopersmith, S. (1967). *The antecedents of self-esteem.* San Francisco: W. H. Freeman and Co.

DeNil, L. F. and Brutten, G. J. (1991). Speech-associated attitudes of stuttering and non-stuttering children. *Journal of Speech and Hearing Research, 34,* 60-66.

Faber, A., & Mazlish, E. (1980). *How to talk so kids will listen and listen so kids will talk.* New York: Avon Books.

Gregory, H.H. (1991). Therapy for elementary school-age children. *Seminars in Speech and Language, 12,* 323-335.

Gregory, H.H. & Campbell, J.H. (1988). Stuttering in the school-age child. In Yoder, D.E. & Kent, R. D. (Eds.), *Decision making in speech-language pathology.* Toronto: Decker.

Kagan, J. (1981). *The second year: The emergence of self-awareness.* Cambridge, MA: Harvard University Press.

Manning, W.H. (1996). *Clinical decision making in the diagnosis and treatment of fluency disorders.* Albany, New York: Delmar Publishers.

Murphy, W. (1996). Empowering children who stutter: Reducing shame, guilt, and anxiety. Annual meeting of the Illinois Speech and Hearing Association, Chicago, IL.

Ramig, P. and Bennett, E. (1995). Working with 7-12 year old children who stutter: Ideas for intervention in the public schools. *Language, Speech, and Hearing Services in Schools, 26,* 138-150.

Shapiro, D. A. (1999). *Stuttering intervention.* Austin, TX: Pro-Ed.

Van Riper, C. (1982). *The nature of stuttering, 2nd edition.* Englewood Cliffs, NJ: Prentice-Hall.

Williams, D. (1985). Talking with children who stutter. In J. Fraser (Ed.), *Counseling stutterers.* Memphis, TN: Stuttering Foundation of America.

Additional Readings and Resources

Andrews, G. and Cutler, J. (1974). Stuttering therapy: The relationship between changes in symptom level and attitudes. *Journal of Speech and Hearing Disorders, 39,* 312-319.

Battle, J. (1994). *Promoting self-esteem, achievement, and well being: An effective instructional curriculum for all levels.* Edmonton, Alberta: James Battle and Associates.

Bajina, K. (1995). Covert aspects associated with the 'stuttering syndrome': Focus on self-esteem. In M. Fawcus (Ed.), *Stuttering: From theory to practice.* London, England: Whurr Publishers Ltd.

Bennett, E.M., Ramig, P.R., and Reveles, V.N. (1993). Speaking attitudes in children: Summer fluency camps. Annual meeting of the American Speech-Language-Hearing Association, Anaheim, CA.

Berkowitz, M., Cook, H., and Haughey, M.J. (1994). A non-traditional fluency program developed for the public school setting. *Language, Speech, and Hearing Services in Schools, 25,* 94-99.

Blood, G. (1995). Power²: Relapse management with adolescents who stutter. *Language, Speech, and Hearing Services in Schools, 26,* 169-179.

Bloodstein, O. (1995). *A handbook on stuttering, 5th ed.* San Diego, CA: Singular Publishing Group, Inc.

Branden, N. (1983). *Honoring the self. The psychology of confidence and respect.* New York: Bantam Books.

Burns, D. (1999). *Feeling good: The new mood therapy.* New York: Avon Books.

Conture, E. G. (1990). *Stuttering, 2nd ed.* Englewood Cliffs, NJ: Prentice-Hall.

Conture, E. G. (1994). The general problem of change. In H. Gregory (Ed.), *Stuttering therapy: Transfer and maintenance.* Memphis, TN: Stuttering Foundation of America.

Cooper, E. B. (1997). Understanding the process. In J. Fraser (Ed.), *Counseling stutterers.* Memphis, TN: Stuttering Foundation of America.

Cooper, E.B. (1976). *Personalized fluency control therapy: An integrated behavior and relationship therapy for stutterers.* Austin, TX: Learning Concepts, Inc.

Crowe, T. A. and Robinson, T. L. (1993). In stuttering: Do we have an ounce to give? *ASHA, 35,* 53-54.

Dell, C. (2005), *Treating the School-Age Child Who Stutters,* 2nd edition, Memphis, TN: Stuttering Foundation of America.

Dinkmeyer, D., McKay, G. D., & Dinkmeyer, J. S. (1989). *Parenting young children.* Circle Pines, MN: American Guidance Service.

Erickson, R. L. (1969). Assessing communicative attitudes among stutterers. *Journal of Speech and Hearing Research, 12,* 711-724.

Fraser, J. (Ed.). (1996). *Therapy for stutterers.* Memphis, TN: Stuttering Foundation of America.

Ginott, H. (1965). *Between parent and child: New solutions to old problems.* New York: Macmillan.

Ginott, H. (1969). *Between parent and teenager.* New York: Macmillan.

Ginott, H. (1972). *Between teacher and child.* New York: Macmillan.

Gregory, H. H. (1987). Handling relapse. Paper presented at Clinical Management of Chronic Stuttering, Washington, D.C.

Gregory, H. H. (1994). Commentary. In J. Fraser (Ed.), *Stuttering therapy: Transfer and maintenance.* Memphis, TN: Stuttering Foundation of America.

Gregory, H. H. & Gregory, C. B. (1999). Counseling children who stutter and their parents. In R. Curlee (Ed.), *Stuttering and related disorders of fluency, 2nd ed.* New York: Thieme Medical Publishers, Inc.

Guitar, B. and Bass, C. (1978). Stuttering therapy: The relation between attitude change and long-term outcome. *Journal of Speech and Hearing Disorders, 15,* 393-400.

Guitar, B. (1999). *Stuttering: An integrated approach to its nature and treatment, 2nd ed.* Baltimore, MD: Williams & Wilkins.

Guitar, Fraser et al. *Therapy in Action: The School-Age Child Who Stutters,* Memphis, TN: Stuttering Foundation of America.

Healey, E. C. & Scott, L. (1995). Strategies for treating elementary school-age children who stutter: An integrated approach. *Language, Speech, and Hearing Services in Schools, 26,* 151-161.

Kelly, E. and Conture, E. (1991). Intervention with school-age stutterers: A parent-child fluency group approach. *Seminars in Speech and Language, 12,* 310-322.

Kelly, E. M., Martin, J. S., Baker, K. E., Rivera, N. I., Bishop, J. E., Krizike, C. B., Stettler, D. S., & Stealy, J. M. (1997). Academic and clinical preparation and practices of school speech language pathologists with people who stutter. *Language, Speech, and Hearing Services in Schools, 28,* 195-212.

LaBlance, G.R., Steckol, K.F., & Smith, V.L. (1994). Stuttering: The role of the classroom teacher. *Teaching Exceptional Children, 26,* 10-12.

Leith, W.R. (1986). Treating the stutterer with atypical cultural influences. In K. O. St. Louis (Ed.), *The atypical stutterer: Principles and practices of rehabilitation.* Orlando, FL: Academic Press.

Luper, H.L., & Mulder, R.L., (1964). *Stuttering: Therapy for children.* Englewood Cliffs, NJ: Prentice-Hall, Inc.

Luterman, D. M. (1991). *Counseling the communicatively disordered and their families, 2nd ed.* Austin, TX: ProEd.

Mallard, A. R. (1991). Using families to help the school-age stutterer: A case study. In L. Rustin (Ed.), *Parents, families and the stuttering child.* San Diego, CA: Singular Publishing Group, Inc.

Manning, W.H. (1991). Making progress during and after treatment. In W. Perkins (Ed.), *Seminars in Speech and Language.* New York: Thieme Medical Publishers.

Matkin, N., Ringle, R., & Snope, T. (1983). Master report of survey discrepancies. In N. Rees & T. Snope (Eds.), *Proceedings of the conference on undergraduate, graduate and continuing education (ASHA Reports No. 13).* Rockville, MD: American Speech-Language-Hearing Association.

McCoy, E. (1992). Bully-proofing your child. *Readers' Digest,* Nov, 199-204.

Nelson, P. (1987). Habits are hard to break. In C. L. Whitefield (Ed.), *Healing the child within: Discovery and recovery for adult children of dysfunctional families.* Pompano Beach, FL: Health Communications.

Perkins, W.H. (1992). *Stuttering prevented.* San Diego, CA: Singular Publishing Group, Inc.

Ramig, P. (2005). *The Child and Adolescent Stuttering Treatment Activity Resource Guide.* New York: Thomson-Delmar.

Ramig, P. R. (1993). Parent-clinician-child partnership in the therapeutic process of the preschool and elementary-aged child who stutters, *Seminars in Speech and Language, 14,* 226-237.

Rustin, L. & Cook, F. (1995). Parental involvement in the treatment of stuttering. *Language, Speech, and Hearing Services in Schools, 26,* 127-137.

Sheehan, J.G. (1994). Relapse and recovery. In J. Fraser (Ed.), *Stuttering therapy: Transfer and maintenance.* Memphis, TN: Stuttering Foundation of America.

Sommers, R.K., and Caruso, A.J. (1995). Inservice training in speech-language pathology: Are we meeting the needs for fluency training? *American Journal of Speech-Language Pathology, 3,* 22-28.

Watson, J.B. (1995). Exploring the attitudes of adults who stutter. *Journal of Communication Disorders, 28,* 143-164.

Wexler, D. (1991). *The prism workbook: A program guide for innovative self-management.* New York: W. W. Norton and Company, Inc.

Zebrowski, P. and Schum, R.L. (1993). Counseling parents of children who stutter. *American Journal of Speech-Language Pathology, 2,* 65-73.

Assessment Scales for Children

Andre, S., & Guitar, B. (1979). The A-19 Scale for children who stutter. In Peters, T., & Guitar, B. (1991). *Stuttering: An integrated approach to its nature and treatment.* Baltimore, MD: Williams & Wilkins and also in (1999) *Stuttering: An integration of contemporary therapies.* Memphis, TN: Stuttering Foundation of America.

Brutten, E., & Shoemaker, D. (1974). Fear survey schedule. In *Southern Illinois Behavior Checklist.* Carbondale, Illinois: Southern Illinois University.

Brutten, E. & Shoemaker, D. (1974). Speech situation checklist. In the *Southern Illinois Checklist.* Carbondale, Illinois. Southern Illinois University. Also, Respond Therapy. DLM Teaching Resources, 1 DLM Park, Allen, Texas 75002.

DeNil, L. & Brutten, G.J (1991). Speech associated attitudes of stuttering and nonstuttering children. *Journal of Speech and Hearing Research, 34,* 60-66.

Devore, J., Nandur, M., & Manning, W. (1984). Projective drawings and children who stutter. *Journal of Fluency Disorders, 9,* 217-226.

Manning, W.H. (1994). The Sea-Scale: Self-efficacy scaling for adolescents who stutter. Paper presented at the annual convention of the American Speech-Language-Hearing Association, New Orleans, LA.

Oyler, M. E. (1996). *Parent perception scale.* Fullerton, CA: Center for Children Who Stutter.

Resources

The Stuttering Foundation
P.O. Box 11749
Memphis, TN. 38111-0749
800-992-9392
www.StutteringHelp.org
www.tartamudez.org
info@StutteringHelp.org

Friends: National Association of Young People Who Stutter
www.friendswhostutter.org

National Stuttering Asssociation
www.nsastutter.org

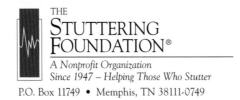

THE
STUTTERING
FOUNDATION®
A Nonprofit Organization
Since 1947 – Helping Those Who Stutter
P.O. Box 11749 • Memphis, TN 38111-0749

www.StutteringHelp.org
www.tartamudez.org

8 tips for teachers

1 Don't tell the student to "slow down" or "just relax."

2 Don't complete words for the student or talk for him or her.

3 Help all members of the class learn to take turns talking and listening. All students — and especially those who stutter — find it much easier to talk when there are few interruptions, and they have the listener's attention.

4 Expect the same quality and quantity of work from the student who stutters as the one who doesn't.

5 Speak with the student in an unhurried way, pausing frequently.

6 Convey that you are listening to the content of the message, not how it is said.

7 Have a one-on-one conversation with the student who stutters about needed accommodations in the classroom. Respect the student's needs, but do not be enabling.

8 Don't make stuttering something to be ashamed of. Talk about stuttering just like any other matter.

Compiled by Lisa A. Scott, Ph.D., The Florida State University
Illustration by Amy L. Dech

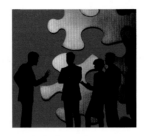

Myths about stuttering

Myth: People who stutter are not smart.

Reality: There is no link whatsoever between stuttering and intelligence.

Myth: Nervousness causes stuttering.

Reality: Nervousness does not cause stuttering. Nor should we assume that people who stutter are prone to be nervous, fearful, anxious, or shy. They have the same full range of personality traits as those who do not stutter.

Myth: Stuttering can be "caught" through imitation or by hearing another person stutter.

Reality: You can't "catch" stuttering. No one knows the exact causes of stuttering, but recent research indicates that family history (genetics), neuromuscular development, and the child's environment, including family dynamics, all play a role in the onset of stuttering.

Myth: It helps to tell a person to "take a deep breath before talking," or "think about what you want to say first."

Reality: This advice only makes a person more self-conscious, making the stuttering worse. More helpful responses include listening patiently and modeling slow and clear speech yourself.

Myth: Stress causes stuttering.

Reality: As mentioned above, many complex factors are involved. Stress is not the cause, but it certainly can aggravate stuttering.